Primary Child and Adolescent Mental Health

T0133871

Primary Child and Adolescent Mental Health

A practical guide
VOLUME III
Second Edition

Dr Quentin Spender
Consultant in Child and Adolescent Psychiatry
Wolverhampton City Primary Care Trust
Wolverhampton, UK

Dr Judith Barnsley
Consultant in Child and Adolescent Psychiatry
Dorset Healthcare University NHS Foundation Trust
Poole, UK

Alison Davies
Primary Mental Health Worker
Sussex Partnership NHS Foundation Trust
Chichester, UK

and

Dr Jenny Murphy
Clinical Psychologist
Dorset Healthcare University NHS Foundation Trust
Poole, UK

Radcliffe Publishing
London • New York

Radcliffe Publishing Ltd
33–41 Dallington Street
London
EC1V 0BB
United Kingdom

www.radcliffepublishing.com

Electronic catalogue and worldwide online ordering facility.

First Edition 2001

British Library Cataloguing in Publication Data

A catalogue record for this book is available from the British Library.

ISBN-13: 978 184619 314 9 (box set)
ISBN-13: 978 184619 544 0 (volume III)

Typeset by KnowledgeWorks Global Ltd, Chennai, India
Printed and bound by Cadmus Communications, USA

Contents

Preface to the second edition

In the decade since the first edition of this book, the way in which mental health services in the United Kingdom are provided to children and adolescents has changed in a number of ways. Although geographical uniformity has proved difficult to achieve, frontline services have been extensively developed to improve the mental health of the under-18 population.

The aim of this book is to give those working at the frontline – the first professionals that a child or parent may meet when asking for help – a practical guide about what to do. The chapters are structured to enable relevant theoretical issues to be summarised simply, followed by detailed suggestions about how to gather relevant information and how to help, leaving referral to specialised services as a last resort.

Our vision is that a whole variety of professionals to whom children or parents may turn for help will have at their fingertips a means of understanding the problems presented, and will be able to offer straightforward ways of helping. Professionals at the frontline need training and advice from more experienced and highly trained colleagues; but we hope this book will also play a role in their professional development and provide an additional source of support, either as a component of learning or as a resource for teaching.

It would be foolhardy not to acknowledge some of the difficulties inherent in providing a universal Child and Adolescent Mental Health Service (CAMHS) that can meet everyone's needs. These barriers include the following.

➤ *Agency cooperation* – Using the broadest definition of CAMHS, services are provided and professionals employed by not only the National Health Service but also by Educational and Social Care organisations; others play a role, such as the youth criminal justice system, substance misuse services and counselling charities. A single child may have contact with a bewildering array of different organisations and individuals, making effective cooperation between them a significant challenge.

➤ *Management issues* – The joint management of Education and Social Care, and the appointment of jointly funded Commissioners, has been introduced to help coordinate the main involved agencies. There remains tremendous variation in management structures. Considering now the narrow definition of CAMHS, specialised services may be part of Mental Health Trusts, Primary Care Trusts or Trusts providing hospital paediatric care. Within these Trusts, specialised CAMHS may be in a directorate with a variety of bedfellows, for instance: adult mental health; adult learning difficulty; community paediatrics; hospital pae-diatrics; health visiting; school nursing; and many others. Some Trusts favour medics in managerial roles such as that of CAMHS Clinical Director; some Trusts prefer non-clinicians for service management roles; others prefer clini-cians such as nurses, psychologists or social workers for both clinical and serv-ice management roles.

➤ This variation in management structures is part of the *'postcode lottery'*, mean-ing that services may be available in one area but not another, and that *where* the child and family live may be as much a factor in determining what help is available as the skill-mix of professionals. Another component of this is that areas of deprivation have higher per capita funding, but in relatively affluent areas, a higher proportion of the population in need may present for help, with the result that services may paradoxically be more stretched in more affluent areas. This can be exacerbated by the cost of housing contributing to difficulties in recruiting staff. The independent sector is just as patchy in its provision (per-haps more). Added to all this is the variation in the four countries of the UK: England, Scotland, Wales and Northern Ireland. We have not attempted in this book to do justice to this, but have stuck to what we know, which is our own practice within three different regions of England: we cannot claim with our limited joint experience to understand the range of service provision within even *one* country.

➤ *Service lacunae* (gaps in what is provided) have persisted, despite a variety of attempts to make services more uniform, such as the National Service Frame-work[1] and the establishment of a peer-reviewing system.[2] An example is the service received by children with learning difficulties and their families, which is still extremely patchy and highly variable.

➤ *Funding issues* – It is beyond the scope of this book to present the arguments about the inequitable share of the funding cake allocated to under-18s com-pared to other age groups, or mental health problems compared to other cat-egories of ill health. Killers such as cancer, heart disease or premature birth are more likely to get the sort of publicity that mobilises political will. Some have described CAMHS as the 'Cinderella of Cinderellas'. Periods of investment tend to be followed by periods of renewed financial stringency. Joint commission-ing arrangements may not be able to prevent huge sums being spent on highly specialised provision for a small number of individuals, thus stifling investment in small-scale outpatient teams: a larger scale preventative approach may be necessary for this.

➤ *Customer confusion* – All of this variation may leave parents very confused about how best to access help for their child. Professionals may also be con-fused about who is best placed to deliver the best help at the best time: the professional who first sees the child may be chosen more by accident than by any logical process. Some acronyms (abbreviations) may add to the overall con-fusion. We give here a selection:

— ABE   Achieving Best Evidence
— ASBO   Antisocial Behaviour Order
— ASSIST   Asylum Seeker Support Initiative Short Term
— BESD   Behavioural, Educational and Social Difficulties
— BEST   Behavioural and Educational Support Team
— BOSS   Business Opportunity Sourcing Service
— BPD   Borderline Personality Disorder
— BPD   Bipolar Disorder
— BPD   Broncho-Pulmonary Dysplasia
— BPS   British Psychological Society
— CAF   Common Assessment Framework
— CAFE   Child and Adolescent Faculty Executive
— CAP   Child and Adolescent Psychiatry
— CORC   CAMHS Outcome Research Consortium
— CPD   Continuing Professional Development
— CPD   Continuous Peritoneal Dialysis
— CPS   Crown Prosecution Service
— CRB   Criminal Records Bureau
— DAT   Drug and Alcohol Team
— DAT   Drug Action Team
— DCSF   Department for Children, Schools and Families
— DNA   Did Not Arrive
— DNA   Deoxyribonucleic acid
— DoH   Department of Health
— DTO   Detention and Training Order
— EBD   Educational and Behavioural Difficulties
— EBPD   Emerging Borderline Personality Disorder
— E2E   Entry to Employment
— FAST   Family Advice and Support Team
— FIP   Family Intervention Project
— FRT   Family Resource Team
— GAP   Guideline Appraisal Panel
— HAVOC   Having an Alternative View of Crime
— HMYOI   Her Majesty's Young Offender Institution
— IRS worker   Integrated Resettlement Support worker
— ISP   Initial Supervision Plan
— ISSP   Intensive Supervision and Surveillance Programme
— JAR   Joint Area Review
— KYPE   Keeping Young People Engaged
— LAC   Looked-After Children
— LD   Learning Difficulty
— MAPPA   Multi-Agency Public Protection Arrangements
— MAST   Multi-Agency Support Team
— MHPW   Mental Health and Psychological Wellbeing
— MLD   Moderate Learning Difficulty

- NEET — Not in Education, Employment or Training
- NHS — National Health Service
- NICE — National Institute for Health and Clinical Excellence
- OFSTED — Office for Standards in Education
- OoH — Out of Hours
- PAYP — Positive Activities for Young People
- PCAMHW — Primary Child and Adolescent Mental Health Worker
- PCSO — Police Community Service Officer
- PCT — Primary Care Trust
- PDP — Personal Development Plan
- PHEW — Psychological Health and Emotional Wellbeing
- PMHW — Primary Mental Health Worker
- PREMs — Patient-Reported Experience Measures
- PROMs — Patient-Reported Outcome Measures
- PRU — Pupil Referral Unit
- PTSD — Post Traumatic Stress Disorder
- PSA — Parenting Support Adviser
- PSR — Pre-Sentence Report
- RAP — Recurrent Abdominal Pain
- RAP — Resource Allocation Panel
- RAP — Resettlement and Aftercare Provision
- RoH — Risk of Harm
- SENCo — Special Educational Needs Coordinator
- SIG — Special Interest Group
- SIPS — Social Inclusion and Pupil Support
- SLA — Service Level Agreement
- SLD — Severe Learning Difficulty
- SMART — Specific, Measurable, Achievable, Realistic and Time-bounded
- SPP — Senior Parenting Practitioner
- SSIW — Social Services Inspectorate for Wales
- TAC — Team Around the Child
- TaMHS — Targeted Mental Health in Schools
- TPU — Teenage Pregnancy Unit
- VLO — Victim Liaison Officer
- WPI — Wales Programme for Improvement
- YADAS — Young Adults' Drug and Alcohol Service
- YIP — Youth Inclusion Programme
- YISP — Youth Inclusion Support Panel
- YJB — Youth Justice Board
- YOI — Young Offender's Institution
- YOIS — Youth Offending Information System
- YOT — Youth Offending Team
- … and many others.

Another change since the first edition of this book is the increasing availability of protocols and guidelines developed to reduce the risks inherent in any dabbling with other people's mental health – and the variability of clinical approach inevitable in a multidisciplinary field. Some are local, others are national, in particular the Scottish Intercollegiate Guideline Network (SIGN)[3] guidelines in Scotland and the National Institute for Health and Clinical Excellence (NICE)[4] guidelines for the whole UK. These aim to make clinical practice more evidence-based and uniform, and should in theory reduce the postcode lottery.

Other developments such as leaflets,[5] information sheets,[6] websites[7] and charities[8] have aimed at reducing the confusion for families of knowing which profession they should go to when, and the confusion for professionals about whether they are duplicating others' work, or alternatively allowing families to fall into the gaps between services. Various ways of combining professionals from different disciplines into teams who are more coordinated, or more convenient for families, or more convenient for agencies, have been devised (see some of the acronyms above), but there seems to be a remarkable lack of uniformity. The Common Assessment Framework[9] is an attempt to save professionals in different agencies from carrying out repeated initial assessments that ask all the same questions: once done by one agency, it should be shared electronically with others who need to be involved. The use of Electronic Health Records is already common in Health Centres, and is due to spread to specialist CAMHS as we write this edition. We anticipate some difficulties including all the information gathered by specialist CAMHS in electronic form – not least because of concerns about who will access the information.

Just as the expectations placed on professionals working in all levels of CAMHS have changed in a decade, so have the lives of young people been transformed by readily available internet access. Social contact can now take place without anyone leaving their rooms. Cyber-bullying and internet grooming (leading to sexual abuse) have added new dimensions to the hazards of adolescent relationships. Whereas previously we might have worried whether we should allow a parent to show us her daughter's diary without permission, we may now be worried about whether to look at a personal blog, and how we should respond to what we may find there. Similarly, whilst there is much helpful information on the Internet, young people can also access unhelpful sites such as pro-anorexia and pro-suicide websites that compound their despair and undermine the help they may be offered or at least need.

One change that has particularly affected the target audience for this book is the advent, at least in some areas, of the Primary Child and Adolescent Mental Health Worker, variously abbreviated as PCAMHW or PMHW. This specialism was just being developed as the first edition was being published. The initial idea for the book (which we must credit to Professor Peter Hill) was as a source of practical information for those working in primary care – the case examples were written with General Practitioners in mind – but GPs may have been only a small proportion of the book's readership. Professor Hill was also part of the group that developed[10] the idea of the Four Tier system and the Primary Child and Adolescent Mental Health Worker (for further details *see* Chapter 1: Context).

The first edition seems to have been devoured by a variety of professionals doing Tier 1 and Tier 2 work, and we hope this edition will cater more overtly for these groups. We have shifted the emphasis to make the book suitable for any profession to whom the Primary Child and Adolescent Mental Health Worker consults. We hope the book will enable frontline practitioners (Tier 1 or universal services) to catch child mental health conditions at an early stage so that interventions can be provided without having to wait for specialised services (Tier 3 or targeted services) to become involved. The authorship, instead of being a mixture of Child and Adolescent Psychiatrists and GPs, is now a mixture of Child and Adolescent Psychiatrists and Primary Child and Adolescent Mental Health Workers.

Rather than tinker with the first edition, we have rewritten the whole book, reorganising some of the chapter structure, but keeping the more successful chapters while updating them. We have persisted in our strategy of breaking-up the text by liberal use of bullet points, tables, case examples, summary boxes (including 'Practice Points' and 'Alarm Bells') and figures. The most striking change is perhaps the first main section of the book (Chapters 2 to 4), which emphasises our developmental approach by describing the differences between three important development stages: pre-school, middle childhood and adolescence. In particular, the chapter on middle childhood contains much of the content of the first chapter in the first edition, which was entitled 'Assessment'. We have also changed the title, to reflect the change in emphasis.

A note on terminology: We have alternated the female and male pronoun when talking about an unspecified child (or parent). We are aware there are various definitions of 'children' (for instance: under-13, Gillick incompetent, under-16 or under-18); 'adolescents' (12–25 being perhaps the most inclusive); and 'young people' (for instance, 16- and 17-year-olds, 11–19 or seven to 25). But we have used these terms colloquially, without attempting to stick to one definition. We have also used the terms 'parent' and 'carer' interchangeably (so as to avoid the cumbersome phrase 'parent or carer'). We have tried to keep abbreviations to a minimum, but have allowed ourselves to use a few, such as: 'CAMHS' for Child and Adolescent Mental Health Services; 'ADHD' for Attention-Deficit/Hyperactivity Disorder; GCSEs for General Certificate of Secondary Education exams; and 'DVDs' for Digital Versatile Discs.

A note on case examples: We have pursued a policy of peppering the text liberally with these, in order to break up the text, maintain clinical relevance and keep things interesting. The case examples vary in their origins: some are based on a single case, with enough details altered to make the identity unrecognisable to anyone but the child and family; some incorporate details of more than one case; and some are fictionalised on the basis of our clinical experience (so effectively incorporating the details of many cases).

We hope that our labours will enable our readers to improve the mental health and emotional well-being of children throughout the United Kingdom, and possibly elsewhere.

Quentin Spender
Judith Barnsley
Alison Davies
Jenny Murphy
April 2011

REFERENCES

1 www.dh.gov.uk/en/Publicationsandstatistics/Publications/PublicationsPolicyAnd Guidance/DH_4089114
2 www.rcpsych.ac.uk/crtu/centreforqualityimprovement/qinmaccamhs.aspx
3 www.sign.ac.uk
4 www.nice.org.uk
5 www.rcpsych.ac.uk
6 CAMHS Evidence Based Practice Unit. *Choosing What's Best For You: what scientists have found helps children and young people who are sad, worried or troubled.* London: CAMHS publications; July 2007. Available at: www.annafreud.org/ebpu (accessed 20 March 2011).
7 www.mentalhealth.org.uk
8 www.youngminds.org.uk
9 www.education.gov.uk/childrenandyoungpeople/strategy/integratedworking/caf/ a0068957/the-caf-process
10 Health Advisory Service. *Together We Stand: the commissioning, role and management of child and adolescent mental health services.* London: HMSO; 1995.

About the authors

Dr Quentin Spender, Consultant in Child and Adolescent Psychiatry, Wolverhampton City Primary Care Trust, Wolverhampton, UK

Dr Judith Barnsley, Consultant in Child and Adolescent Psychiatry, Dorset Healthcare University NHS Foundation Trust, Poole, UK

Alison Davies, Primary Mental Health Worker, Sussex Partnership NHS Foundation Trust, Chichester, UK

Dr Jenny Murphy, Clinical Psychologist, Dorset Healthcare University NHS Foundation Trust, Poole, UK

Acknowledgements

This book germinated from an idea that we must credit to Professor Emeritus Peter Hill, who wanted to fashion a companion volume to the same publisher's *The Child Surveillance Handbook*,[1] of which he was an initial co-author. Along with our own changing co-authorship, we have benefited from the direct or indirect input of the following: Rosemarie Berry, Chrissy Boardman, Teri Boutwood, Nina Bunce, Anna Calver, Esther Crawley, David Candy, Steve Clarke, David Rex, Moira Doolan, Danya Glaser, Gill Goodwillie, Sue Horobin, Amelia Kerswell, Karen King, Sebastian Kraemer, Karen Majors, Rebecca Park, Joanna Pearse, Nigel Speight, Anne Stewart and Wendy Woodhouse. We would also like to thank the children and families whom we have all seen in our clinical work: they have taught us so much, and many of them have provided us with the stories for our case examples.

Note

1 First edition published in 1990, second edition published in 1994 and third edition published in 2009. Hall D, Williams J, Elliman D. *The Child Surveillance Handbook*. 3rd ed. London and New York: Radcliffe Publishing; 2009.

PART 6

Problems that may present at any age

CHAPTER 30

Disorders of conduct

INTRODUCTION

Traditionally, mental health disorders in children and adolescents have been divided into **disorders of conduct** and **disorders of emotion**. Disorders of conduct are behaviours that are seen as problems, such as aggression, fire-setting or stealing; and disorders of emotion are feelings that are seen as problems, such as anxiety, depression or obsessions. The distinction is to some extent an oversimplification.

➤ Most emotions result in observable behaviours, for instance:
  — anxiety can lead to avoidance
  — depression can lead to self-harm
  — obsessions can lead to compulsions.
➤ Many factors may influence both behaviour and emotions, for instance:
  — parental warmth or criticism
  — bullying
  — success in sport or academic work.
➤ If you scrape the surface of a child behaving badly, you are likely to find more than a few emotions lurking underneath, concealed to a greater or lesser extent by the behaviour.

One way to understand this better is to view **behaviour as a form of communication**. Ask yourself what the child may be expressing in behaviour that he is not expressing in other ways. There may (for instance) be reasons for his not expressing feelings in words: lack of a language for emotions, expressive language delay, no one to listen, or simply that the feelings are too difficult to acknowledge or to express directly.

Another oversimplification is that bad behaviour is *all* due to bad parenting. On the contrary, the earlier behaviour problems start, the more likely there are to be underlying biological factors; the later they start, the more likely they are to be influenced by peers; although in both cases, parenting style can have a big influence (*see* Box 30.3 below). Two broad groups have been described: the early-onset group, who tend to have conduct problems persisting throughout their life course, starting with preschool challenging behaviour, progressing through delinquency in adolescence, and continuing into antisocial personality disorder in adults; and the adolescent-onset group, who tend to grow out of their conduct problems by the end of their teens.[1]

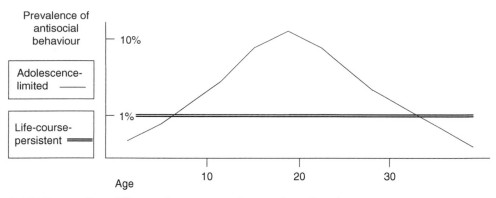

FIGURE 30.1 Two different time courses for conduct disorder

It is in the early onset group that biological problems can be missed: the behaviour is everyone's main concern, social circumstances may be dire, and the parents may themselves be struggling with various sorts of adversity (they may have had similar biological problems as children, with mental health consequences in the present). Examples of conditions with a strong biological component that are commonly associated with behaviour problems, and are likely to make them more severe and start earlier, are shown in Box 30.1. The importance of identifying these in the early onset group is that they are likely to prevent or dilute the success of any treatment if not identified.

BOX 30.1 Factors associated with early-onset behaviour problems that have a strong biological component

ADHD
Impaired hearing
Language disorder
Dyspraxia (developmental motor coordination difficulties)
Specific literacy difficulties (dyslexia)
Autistic spectrum disorder
Other family traits that probably have a genetic component:
- parental criminality
- impulse control problems
- callous-unemotional traits

There are many other risk factors for the development of antisocial behaviour.[2] Box 30.2 shows some psychosocial factors, divided into those intrinsic to the child, those in the child's immediate environment, and those in the child's wider environment. Many of these often act together for an individual child.

BOX 30.2 Psychosocial risk factors for the development of antisocial behaviour

CHILD CHARACTERISTICS:
- *Difficult temperament* from birth – in the developmental history, ask about how the child fed, slept and cried in the first year.
- *Attributional bias* – a tendency to perceive neutral acts by others as hostile.
- *Callous and unemotional traits* – not appearing to appreciate the feelings of others or the consequences of actions.

IMMEDIATE ENVIRONMENT:[3]
- *Postnatal depression* – this seems to be a common finding in the developmental history. It is related to difficult temperament in a chicken-and-egg way (the child's temperament may influence, and be influenced by, the mother's mood).
- *Child-rearing practices* – antisocial behaviour has been shown to be linked to five factors:
  - lack of positive reinforcement and warmth;
  - lack of parental involvement;
  - poor parental supervision and monitoring of the child's behaviour;
  - harsh or inconsistent discipline, or hostility directed at the child;
  - defective problem-solving.
- *Parent-child interaction patterns* – studies of moment-to-moment patterns of interaction in families of antisocial children show that children are inadvertently trained to persist with disruptive behaviour if:
  - this gets them more attention (even if this is angry or irritable attention) than pro-social behaviours
  - this gets them out of having to do something they don't want to do
  - this enables them to get their own way more often.

CHILD ABUSE:
All four forms of abuse can present with behaviour problems.
- *Neglect* – some children *have* to misbehave, in order to get any attention.
- *Physical abuse* – a child who has been the victim of violence may react in either of two extreme ways: by becoming withdrawn and helpless; or by becoming aggressive or violent himself ('identification with the aggressor' – modelling the abuser's behaviour).
- *Emotional abuse* is the hardest to define, but overlaps with some of the child-rearing practices and interaction patterns described above. *Domestic violence* is one example of emotional abuse which often goes unrecognised, and from which the effects on children are often underestimated. For instance, a child may be very distressed by watching his mother being beaten up by his father, but may later copy this aggressive behaviour. Some children may also be victims of domestic violence, i.e. physical abuse.
- *Sexual abuse* may lead to the emergence of behaviour problems in girls or boys who were previously free of such problems. Any pattern of behavioural or emotional disorder can be caused by child sexual abuse.

Any **losses** that may be important for the child, such as:
- an important father-figure leaving
- moving house
- moving schools
- the death of a nurturing grandparent
- the death of a pet.

WIDER ENVIRONMENT:
- *School factors* affect behaviour problems independently of home background, particularly if they are unfriendly, poorly organized, have low staff morale and have poor communication between staff and parents.
- *Wider social influences*, such as overcrowding, poor housing, a lack of social supports and a crime-ridden neighbourhood are strongly associated with childhood antisocial behaviour. It is not clear whether this is all due to the immediate environmental factors discussed above, or whether they have an independent effect: probably both.
- *Gangs* of young people, of varying ages and both sexes, can be a particular problem in some areas, usually urban, where loyalties between members of the same gang transcend parental values, legal sanctions and common sense, leading to groups behaving in a way that most of the constituent individuals probably would not – in some extreme cases committing group rape or murder.
- *Cultural and ethnic issues* have a complex interaction with all child mental health problems. The impact on the child varies between different ethnic groups, cultural backgrounds, and degrees of assimilation into the surrounding culture.

There is a tendency for professionals to focus on deficits in parenting, so it is always worth having another look at the characteristics of the child: considering all those possibilities mentioned in Box 30.1 and the top section of Box 30.2. One characteristic that is in the transition phase from hot research topic to clinical applicability is the temperamental attribute of having callous and unemotional traits, which may have significant genetic and biological components. Children in this sub-group may:[4]
➤ show little if any remorse or empathy
➤ be less likely to have comorbid emotional disorders
➤ show a form of aggression that is cold rather than passionate, and instrumental rather than reactive
➤ be more difficult to parent – their behaviour seems less related to parenting attributes
➤ respond less well to punishment, even time-out. They do respond as well as other children to positive parenting, including rewards
➤ have difficulty recognising facial expressions, particularly those showing fear
➤ look less at the eyes in faces – and be more able to recognise facially expressed emotions when asked to look at the eyes
➤ be perpetrators of bullying
➤ be more likely to develop severe delinquency, aggression and criminal behaviour.

The clinical implications of this are that behaviour management for parents of these children needs to be tailored to their needs (for instance, by advocating less time-out and more rewards); and the children may benefit from help in recognising others' and their own emotional states, for instance by being trained to look at the eyes in faces, or having a review at the end of each day with a carer about the emotionally salient events of the day.

DEFINITIONS

Antisocial behaviour can be regarded as a ***disorder*** if there is *impairment* as well as behaviour that adults don't like. Examples of adverse consequences of antisocial behaviour include escalations of conflict within the home, management difficulties for the school teacher, and friendship difficulties: these are examples of

BOX 30.3 Behaviours seen in conduct disorder

Excessive fighting, with frequent initiation of fights
Deliberate and repeated destruction of others' property
Lying to obtain goods or favours or to avoid obligations
Repeated stealing outside the home without confrontation, e.g. shoplifting
Stealing while confronting a victim, e.g. purse-snatching, mugging
Using a weapon that can cause serious physical harm to others, e.g. a bat, brick, broken bottle, knife or gun
Breaking into someone else's house, building or car
Frequent truancy from school, beginning before thirteen years
Often bullying, threatening or intimidating others
Running away from home at least twice overnight, or once for more than a single night – unless this was to avoid physical or sexual abuse
Often staying out after dark, despite parental prohibition, beginning before 13 years
Demonstrates physical cruelty to other people, e.g. ties up, cuts or burns a victim
Cruelty to animals
Deliberate fire-setting, with a risk or intention of causing serious damage
Forcing another person into sexual activity against their wishes

BOX 30.4 Behaviours seen in oppositional defiant disorder

Unusually frequent and severe temper tantrums for the child's developmental level
Argues often with adults
Often actively refuses adults' requests or defies rules
Often deliberately annoys people
Often blames others for his or her mistakes or behaviour
Is often touchy or easily annoyed by others
Is often angry or resentful
Is often spiteful or vindictive

impairment. Behaviour problems sufficient to cause some impairment are common, affecting approximately 5% of children and 10% of adolescents. They are commoner in urban than rural areas.

Conduct disorder is a psychiatric term, which simply implies having more than three of the behaviours shown in Box 30.3.[5] A milder and earlier form is called **oppositional-defiant disorder**: there should be at least four of the features shown in Box 30.4.[6] Although these are technically diagnoses, the terms do not contribute any understanding of what is going on for the child, as for instance diagnostic terms such as ADHD or dyslexia or Asperger's disorder might. Some practitioners prefer to avoid using these terms altogether, for fear that the labels will be seen as implying a medical disorder intrinsic to the child, and misused by parents as an excuse for inaction or a means of obtaining Disability Living Allowance. For instance, a diagnosis of oppositional defiant disorder should lead to each parent thinking about how to respond to the child differently, and perhaps attending a behaviour management group – but if it leads to a parent locating the problem entirely within the child and not wishing to change anything, then it is probably counterproductive.

Oppositional defiant disorder and conduct disorder can get easily confused with ADHD (*see* Chapter 31). Although they often occur together, they are conceptually different, and have different implications for management, as shown in simplified form in Table 30.1.

TABLE 30.1 Differentiating ADHD from the two other disruptive behaviour disorders

	ADHD	**Oppositional defiant disorder or conduct disorder**
Epidemiology	ICD-10: 1–2% DSM-IV: 3–5% male/female 4:1	5% male/female 4:1
Aetiology	Mainly biological: genetic and neurodevelopmental	Mainly environmental: social context and details of parenting
Contexts	Home and school	Can be in only one setting
Age	Symptoms start before the age of seven; diagnosis should ideally be made in the second year of school	Antisocial behaviour can be apparent from nursery school onwards
Symptoms	Inattention Hyperactivity Impulsivity	Non-compliance Aggression Other antisocial actions
Treatment	Stimulant medication (large amount of evidence) Behaviour management School management	Environmental manipulation Behaviour management training (easiest under eight; most difficult in adolescence)

There are clear continuities in behaviour. Aggression, for instance, is remarkably persistent over time (*see* Chapter 17). Preschool behaviour problems (oppositionality, defiance and tantrums) above the norm are likely to continue into middle childhood and adolescence, taking a slightly different form at each stage. The preschooler who tantrums and won't comply may become the disruptive primary school child with academic failure, the teenager whose behaviour breaks the law (a delinquent), and the adult with an antisocial personality and continuing criminal behaviour. In contrast, antisocial behaviour arising for the first time in adolescence is more likely to subside. Because of this clear developmental trajectory, it is dangerous to say of difficult preschoolers: 'He'll grow out of it'. Some will, but usually only because their parents find effective ways of coping with the behaviour.

ASSESSMENT

Assessment can be based around the *four-P grid* described in Chapter 6 on Risk and Resilience (Table 6.3). The case example illustrates how the grid can be used.

BOX 30.5 Behaviours seen in conduct disorder

When he is six years old, Christopher's teacher asks the social inclusion pupil support worker to get involved because of Christopher's disruptive behaviour at school.

The social inclusion pupil support worker meets with Christopher's mother, who tells her that Christopher is difficult also at home, often losing his temper and shouting at the rest of his family (mother and four-year-old sister). Christopher's mother discloses that she was depressed after his birth. As a baby, he was very demanding; he cried a lot, especially in the evenings, until he was about seven months old; he wouldn't feed well, and he couldn't seem to sleep much at night. Christopher's father left when he was three years old, and there has been no more than intermittent contact since. Christopher then went to nursery school every morning, but found it difficult to separate. He had the same problem initially in the reception class, but settled with support from a teaching assistant, who unfortunately could not transfer with him up to Year 1. That school year actually got off to a bad start because he missed the first two weeks with a persistent ear infection, and his mother recalls thinking that he had some difficulty hearing things for a few weeks after that. The social inclusion pupil support worker plots some contributory factors in the four-P grid as a way of understanding Christopher's situation more thoroughly (*see* Table 30.2).

The social inclusion pupil support worker gets Christopher to join some after-school activities. He particularly enjoys football, karate and drama. As a result, Christopher's mother has more time available to chat to other parents at the school gates (her daughter is no trouble). She also joins some of their weekend social activities. She agrees with the social inclusion pupil support worker's suggestion of joining a behaviour management group for parents. There she learns to play with Christopher more, praise him more often, spot his good side, and spend less time telling him what not to do. The social inclusion pupil support worker negotiates with the special needs coordinator at the school for Christopher to be put on the special needs register and have some extra help in class for his reading. Although it is only three hours per week, this extra help in literacy seems to help Christopher manage his behaviour. At home, both Christopher and his mother lose their tempers less and start enjoying each other's company more. Unfortunately, Christopher's father continues to be rather haphazard in his contact arrangements, and refuses to get involved with the parenting group or meeting staff from school.

TABLE 30.2 Four-P grid applied to Case Example 30.5

	Biological	**Psychological**	**Social**
Predisposing (Vulnerability factors)	Postnatal depression	Difficult temperament	Absent father
Precipitating (Trigger factors)	Missed the beginning of Year 1 due to an ear infection	Less support from teaching assistants in the classroom	Going from Reception to Year 1 at school
Perpetuating (Maintaining factors)	Christopher is struggling to learn to read	Christopher's mother sees him very negatively (like his father)	Social isolation
Protective (Resilience)	Mother's depression has been adequately treated	Mother keen to join a parenting group	Mother wants to meet new parents

Filling in some or all of the boxes on the four-P grid can help you think about the variety of factors contributing to the child's presenting problem, and summarise the current predicament in a way that can lead on to management options. If you are stuck about what to do, the best place to start will be the protective factors, so it is worth looking hard for these.

There are two essential components that should always be included in an assessment: the *developmental history* and the *family history*; initially, these may not need to be in much detail, since further information can be added later.

The *developmental history* does not mean simply reciting all the milestones in the parent-held health record (red book), although it is important to know about any form of developmental delay or significant medical problem. For an older teenager, it may be sufficient at first meeting to know whether she has gone to a mainstream or a special school and whether she has had any special needs help. A fuller developmental history can be extremely helpful with younger children, and should cover anything that might have affected the developing relationship between the child and main caregivers, for instance (*see* Box 30.2):

➤ postnatal depression: mothers are usually quite open to a question about this
➤ Infant temperament: how was she as a baby? How was feeding and sleeping? Did she cry a lot?
➤ domestic violence, or conflict between parents who are about to separate; this sort of turmoil often seems to coincide with a worsening of the child's behaviour

➤ loss of a main caring figure, through death or separation
➤ any form of abuse
➤ social factors such as difficult neighbours or overcrowded living conditions
➤ cultural or ethnic issues.

A brief *family history* should include questions such as:
➤ Who else is living in the same household?
➤ Who and where are any siblings or half-siblings?
➤ Who if anyone supports the main caregiver, such as grandparents?
➤ Have there been any significant deaths or other losses recently?
➤ What is the pattern of contact (in cases of parental separation) with the absent parent?
➤ Is there anyone else in the family who is similar to the child or who had similar problems as a child?

MANAGEMENT

Behaviour problems seen in preschool and primary school children

The commonest behaviours which parents complain about in preschool children are sleeping difficulties (*see* Chapter 36); feeding difficulties (*see* Chapter 16); hyperactivity (*see* Chapter 31); and tantrums, aggression and sibling rivalry (*see* Chapter 17).[7] Techniques that can be applied to non-compliance in general are described in Chapter 13 on Behaviour Management.

Behaviour problems in the 11-18s

These are generally more difficult to treat. Those with the most severe conduct disorders tend also to be law-breakers, which means that, from the perspective of the criminal justice system, they are thought of as delinquents. The definition of a *juvenile delinquent* in the UK is a person between the ages of 10 and 17 years inclusive who has committed an offence which would be criminal in an adult. Thus the definition is legal, and not directly related to mental health.

As mentioned in the introductory paragraph of this chapter, there are two groups of delinquents:
➤ those whose offending starts and ends in adolescence
➤ those whose conduct disorder has started in early or middle childhood, whose offending tends to persist beyond adolescence, and who are at risk of developing antisocial personality disorder in adulthood.

The first group could be regarded as experimenting and rebelling, in a way that most adolescents have to do as part of their development. If there are harmful consequences, then these young people may need help, for instance from Youth Offending Teams or Substance Misuse Teams.

The second group are more likely to have associated mental health problems, special educational needs and social problems severe enough to warrant the involvement of social services.

What is the role of Tier 1 professionals in delinquency?

Once delinquency is established, it becomes much more difficult to intervene effectively. Important early interventions include:

➤ improving the parenting skills of carers of children under eight years old (*see* Chapter 13)[8]

➤ detecting specific and generalised learning difficulties, and ensuring that children with such special educational needs receive the help they need (*see* Chapter 35)

➤ detecting ADHD from the second year of primary school onwards, and providing appropriate recognition of the child's difficulties and an applicable treatment package (*see* Chapter 31)

➤ recognising all forms of abuse and stopping the abuse from continuing (*see* Chapter 12)

➤ a highly structured home-visiting programme to young low-income, first-time mothers by health visitors[9]

➤ providing high-quality nursery education for all preschool children. Long-term studies have shown a reduction in offending behaviour in adolescence – as well as many other positive outcomes – amongst groups of children whose preschool experience has been enriched in this way.[10,11] The economic returns of early childhood interventions exceed cost by an average ratio of six to one: programmes must be highly structured and focused on the most vulnerable families[12]

➤ recognising autistic spectrum disorders and ensuring that parents and teacher understand the ways in which such children are different from their peers and need modifications of their environment (*see* Chapter 32).

Can established delinquency be treated?

Treating established delinquency is becoming increasingly possible. Effective interventions include Multisystemic Therapy, Multidimensional Treatment Foster Care and Functional Family Therapy.[13] All three of these are currently undergoing trials in the UK. The components of Multisystemic Therapy are shown in Box 30.6.[14]

BOX 30.6 Components of multi-systemic therapy

These include:

- family therapy which focuses on effective communication, taking a problem-solving approach to day-to-day conflicts and instituting predictable rewards and sanctions
- encouragement to spend more time with peers who do not have problems, and to stop seeing other delinquents
- liaison with school to improve learning and homework performance, and restructure after-school hours
- individual development, including assertiveness training against negative peer influences
- empowerment of young people and their parents to cope with family, school, peer and neighbourhood problems. The emphasis is on promoting the family's own problem-solving abilities, not providing ready-made answers.

Coordination with other agencies, such as juvenile justice, social services, and education.

As its name implies, this addresses the various systems or contexts in which the adolescent's behaviour takes place: the family, school, the friendship group, the adolescent's own internal world, and any other agencies involved. Although it is very labour intensive, with each therapist having only a small caseload and requiring extensive training and supervision, Multisystemic Therapy has been shown to be cost-effective, as it reduces offending rates and can have other positive outcomes, thus saving some of the money otherwise spent in the courts, on institutional care and on fostering.

Multidimensional Treatment Foster Care is recommended for young people aged 13–18 years already in foster care, or close to going into care. It is another example of a multi-component treatment and includes:

➤ training foster care families in behaviour management and providing a supportive family environment

➤ providing a behavioural framework for the young person. This should allow the young person to earn privileges (such as time on the computer and extra telephone time with friends) when engaging in positive living and social skills (for example, being polite and making her bed) and good behaviour at school.

➤ individual problem-solving skills training for the young person

➤ family therapy for the birth parents in order to provide a supportive environment for the young person to return to after treatment.[15]

Functional Family Therapy is described in Chapter 8 on Family Issues.

REFERRAL

This depends so much on local circumstances that it is difficult to generalise. Distinguish between the antisocial behaviour and the associated problems; between pre-adolescent and adolescent. For pre-adolescents, the behaviour may indicate referral to a parent-training group, but it is important to consider the conditions in Box 30.1. For adolescents, it may be possible to refer to the preventive arm of the local Youth Offending Team, but it is still important to consider associated conditions (such as those in Box 30.7). One of the commonest of these to be missed is depression (*see* Chapter 26), which is often difficult to diagnose if it is concealed by the behaviour.

BOX 30.7 Conditions that may be associated with antisocial behaviour in adolescents

Depression
ADHD
Specific literacy difficulties (dyslexia)
Autistic spectrum disorder
Substance misuse
Post-traumatic stress disorder (for instance, following abuse)
Bereavement reaction

BOX 30.8 Case Example

Andrea is 14 years old when she is placed in a children's home because three successive sets of foster parents have found her behaviour too difficult to manage. She sets fire to the contents of the waste bin in her room, but calls for help after five minutes. A member of staff at the home extinguishes the fire with only minor damage to some of her belongings, her bedding and the decorations in her room.

Because of the presence of other young people in the home, the police take the episode very seriously and charge Andrea with arson. The court requests an assessment by the Youth Offending Team and the Looked-After Children Team.

The psychologist working for the Looked-After Children Team sees Andrea alone and with her social worker. It emerges that Andrea was sexually abused by one of her mother's partners, and is still furious with her mother for not protecting her. The day before Andrea set fire to her waste bin, her mother failed to keep a promised visit. Another stressor to emerge is that Andrea missed several months of schooling due to her frequent changes of carer, and has not yet started her Year 10 work, although it is already November. She has recently been turned down for the school of her choice, close to her children's home.

The Youth Offending Team worker discusses with Andrea her offending behaviour. She has previously stolen things from shops, and has been involved in some fights in one of her schools, but this episode of arson is her first serious offence. Andrea says she never intended to cause any significant damage, but merely wanted to burn some letters from her mother in her waste bin. She thought she would be able to put the fire out herself with a blanket, but this didn't work, so she panicked and called for help. Before one of the staff of the children's home could get the fire extinguisher to Andrea's room and get it to work, the fire did some further damage, which Andrea states she had not intended.

The Crown Court judge takes into account both reports, and commutes the expected custodial sentence to 100 hours of community service and a one-year Supervision Order.

Andrea has to move to a new children's home, but is accepted by a school near there and at last begins her Year 10 studies. She gets help from the special needs department at her new school to catch up with her GCSE coursework. She has weekly sessions with her Youth Offending Team worker, who discusses with her the relationship between her offending behaviour and her feelings about her past abuse. Her community service involves a gardening project, linked with the development of a new outdoor playground. Unfortunately, she still cannot establish regular contact with anyone from her family of origin. Nevertheless, Andrea cooperates to a greater extent with the staff of her new children's home, as she feels they understand the kind of difficulties she has to cope with. She does not start any more fires.

BOX 30.9 Case Example

David is 10 years old when he is permanently excluded from school for repeated fights in the playground and swearing at a teacher. He is given a place in a Pupil Referral Unit, where his behaviour settles.

The community school nurse discusses his difficulties with the primary mental health worker. David has a family background of domestic violence, and was on the Child Protection Register as a three-year-old because of this. His mother does not currently have a partner, but there are four other children at home, two older than David and two younger. Staff members at the Pupil Referral Unit debate whether to reintegrate him to a mainstream school or keep him in a special school environment.

The primary mental health worker meets with David's mother, who says she is really not sure how to manage his violent outbursts of behaviour. She recalls a difficult temperament from birth. His behaviour became more challenging around the time when his father was violent to her: David's mother persuaded his father to leave when he was three. Staff at his nursery repeatedly discussed with her their concerns about David's behaviour, which mother now thinks was connected to all the disruption at home. He seemed to settle in reception and Year 1, when the family situation was more stable. In Year 2, mother had a new boyfriend, with whom she had two more children; he has since left the family home. David did not get on well with this man, and resented the arrival of his two younger half-siblings. His behaviour became progressively more difficult for the primary school staff to manage, although they helped him in various ways, including a few hours per week of a learning support assistant; they also involved the social inclusion pupil support worker and school educational psychologist. David's mother does not want a referral to specialist CAMHS.

The primary mental health worker speaks to David's special needs coordinator, who explains that his behaviour is easy to manage in the small classes of the Pupil Referral Unit; the school uses a behavioural system focused very much on rewards for any good behaviour or academic achievement. However, he really struggles with his reading and spelling, and is only just beginning to write with joined-up letters.

At a multi-professional meeting that includes David's mother, it is agreed that he would be unlikely to cope with a mainstream school environment. It is decided to put him forward for a full assessment of educational needs, on the grounds of his behaviour and his specific literacy difficulties. The educational psychologist agrees to support this.

David's subsequent Statement of Educational Needs names a special school for behavioural, emotional and social difficulties. He finds this much easier to cope with than his mainstream primary school. No attempts are made to integrate him into mainstream secondary school. He makes slow but steady progress with his writing, reading and spelling.

RESOURCE: FURTHER READING FOR PROFESSIONALS

• Matthys W, Lochman JE. *Oppositional Defiant Disorder and Conduct Disorder in Children.* Oxford: Wiley-Blackwell; 2009.

REFERENCES

1 Moffitt TE. Adolescence-limited and life-course-persistent antisocial behavior: a developmental taxonomy. *Psychological Review.* 1993; **100**(4): 674–701.
2 Goodman R, Scott S. *Child Psychiatry.* 2nd ed. Oxford: Wiley-Blackwell; 2005.
3 Patterson GR, Reid JB, Dishion TJ. *Antisocial Boys.* Eugene, OR: Castalia; 1992.
4 Dadds MR, Rhodes T. Aggression in young children with concurrent callous-unemotional traits: can the neurosciences inform progress and innovation in treatment approaches? *Philos Trans R Soc Lond B Biol Sci.* 2008; **363**(1503): 2567–76.
5 Spender Q, Scott S. Management of antisocial behaviour in childhood. *Advances in Psychiatric Treatment.* 1997; **3**: 128–37.
6 Both boxes are adapted from a combination of ICD-10 (World Health Organization. *The ICD-10 Classification of Mental and Behavioural Disorders: diagnostic criteria for research.* Geneva: World Health Organization; 1993) and DSM-IV (American Psychiatric Association. *Diagnostic and Statistical Manual of Mental Disorders.* Washington, DC: American Psychiatric Association; 1994). The conduct disorder behaviours are sorted roughly in the order they most commonly present.
7 Hall DMB, Hill P, Elliman D. *The Child Surveillance Handbook.* 3rd ed. Oxford: Radcliffe Publishing; 2009.
8 National Institute for Health and Clinical Excellence. *Parent-training/Education Programmes in the Management of Children with Conduct Disorders* [Technology Appraisal Guidance 102]. London: NICE; 2006. Available at: www.nice.org.uk/TA102 (accessed 1 April 2011).
9 www.iscfsi.bbk.ac.uk/projects/nurse-family-partnership-implementation-evaluation
10 Schweinhart LJ. Crime prevention by the High/Scope Perry Preschool Program. *Victims and Offenders.* 2007; **2**(2): 141–60.
11 Reynolds AJ, Temple JA, Robertson DL, *et al.* Long-term effects of an early childhood intervention on educational achievement and juvenile arrest: a 15-year follow-up of low-income children in public schools. *JAMA.* 2001; **285**(18): 2339–46.
12 National Institute for Health and Clinical Excellence. *Antisocial Personality Disorder: treatment, management and prevention* [Clinical Guideline 77]. London: NICE; 2009. Available at: www.nice.org.uk/CG77 (accessed 1 April 2011).
13 Ibid.
14 Goodman, op. cit.
15 National Institute for Health and Clinical Excellence, 2009, op. cit.

CHAPTER 31

Developmental disorders, Part 1: Attention deficit hyperactivity disorder

INTRODUCTION

The term *developmental disorders* is used to refer to a group of conditions in which the key features are due to problems with development in one or more areas. The degree of abnormality, or difference from the norm, varies hugely, so these problems are often described as existing along a *spectrum* – where 'normal' is at one end and a clear disorder (such as autism) is at the other end: in-between there is variation in the number of features present and their severity.

The most common developmental disorders are:

➤ attention deficit hyperactivity disorder (ADHD) – covered in this chapter
➤ autistic spectrum disorders (ASD) – *see* Chapter 32
➤ language disorders – *see* Chapter 33
➤ dyspraxia (developmental motor coordination disorder) – *see* Chapter 34
➤ specific learning difficulties (such as dyslexia, dysgraphia or dyscalculia) – *see* Chapter 35.

These overlap, so it is not uncommon for an individual child to have more than one developmental disorder, as shown in Figure 31.1, although one may be the most apparent or causing the most difficulties.

All developmental disorders are more common in children with learning difficulties and in boys. The gender difference in ADHD, for instance, is less in community samples (boys to girls 4:1) than clinic samples of referrals (10:1), perhaps because they tend to present differently, with more prominent inattention and less prominent hyperactivity in girls.[1]

Prevalence of attention and concentration problems and ADHD

Reported prevalence rates vary, according to the country, sample studied, methodology and definitions used. Between 3–9% of school aged children in the UK and about 2% of adults worldwide will meet the DSM-IV criteria for ADHD; 1–2% meet the stricter ICD-10 diagnostic criteria for hyperkinetic disorder (HKD).[2] Many more children (up to 20%) have difficulties with attention and concentration, as shown in Figure 31.2.[3]

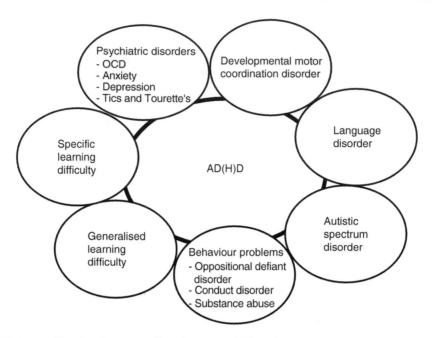

FIGURE 31.1 Overlap between Developmental Disorders

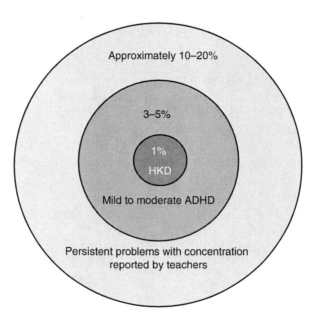

FIGURE 31.2 Rates of different causes of inattention

ASSESSMENT

The key features of ADHD are:
➤ inattention
➤ hyperactivity
➤ impulsivity.

These should be *pervasive* (occurring in different settings such as home and school) and *cause significant impairment in functioning* (such as academic underachievement, impulsive risk-taking or difficulty sustaining relationships with others). In later adolescence and adult life, the range of possible impairments includes:
➤ educational and occupational underachievement
➤ accident-proneness
➤ difficulties in making and keeping friends
➤ substance misuse
➤ criminal activity
➤ difficulties in organising daily activities
➤ dangerous driving
➤ difficulties in managing childcare
➤ difficulties in maintaining intimate relationships.

For a child to be diagnosed with ADHD, he should have a minimum number from each of two (DSM-IV) or three (ICD-10) groups of symptoms (*see* below), combined with at least a moderate degree of psychological, social and/or educational impairment. It is essential to compare the child's behaviour to a normal child of the same developmental age. Many two and three year olds are normally overactive with a short attention span – this does not mean they have a disorder. It is easier to make judgements of the criteria in children over the age of four years. Other possible reasons why the child may be having difficulties paying attention need also to be considered (*see* Box 31.1).

BOX 31.1 Reasons (other than ADHD) why children may have difficulty paying attention

Developmental reasons
Unrecognised learning difficulties, specific or general (*see* Chapter 35)
Language disorder (*see* Chapter 33)
Autistic spectrum disorder (*see* Chapter 32)
High IQ (gifted children may get bored or switch off in class)

Emotional reasons
Depression (*see* Chapter 26)
Anxiety (*see* Chapter 20)
Trauma – being a victim of bullying, other abuse, a natural disaster or being a refugee
    (*see* Chapter 37)
Other worries – being preoccupied with something else
Significant attachment difficulties (*see* Chapter 7)

Social reasons
Drug and alcohol abuse
Domestic violence
Parental substance misuse or criminality

Pharmacological reasons
Non-prescribed medications
Prescribed medications, such as anticonvulsants, antihistamines or benzodiazepines

As a diagnosis of ADHD is made by satisfying enough criteria on a list, ADHD may coexist with one or more of the conditions in Box 31.1, and it often does, as shown in Figure 31.1 and discussed further below (under 'the problem of comorbidity').

The two main symptom lists used are the *International Classification of Mental and Behavioural Disorders, 10th revision* (ICD-10)[4] and the *Diagnostic and Statistical Manual of Mental Disorders, 4th edition* (DSM-IV).[5] Box 31.2 shows a synopsis of the ICD-10 criteria for hyperkinetic disorder, which has a narrower definition than the DSM-IV category of ADHD. The criterion of a clear beginning to symptoms before the age of seven years has been deliberately omitted, as a late onset does not imply any differences in other characteristics of the condition.[6]

BOX 31.2 ICD-10: diagnostic criteria for hyperkinetic disorder

The child should have six or more of the following nine symptoms of **inattention**:
● Failure to give close attention to detail, so making careless mistakes
● Difficulty concentrating on tasks or play activities
● Failure to listen when spoken to directly
● Failure to follow through on instructions and finish tasks
● Lack of organisation
● Reluctance to start tasks that require concentration
● Tendency to lose items necessary for tasks
● Distraction by irrelevant activity
● Forgetfulness in daily activities.

The child should have three or more of the following five symptoms of **hyperactivity**:
● Fidgets
● Unable to stay seated
● Inappropriate running or climbing
● Noisiness
● Being 'on the go' or often acting as if 'driven by a motor'.

The child should have one or more of the following four symptoms of **impulsivity**:
● Tendency to blurt out answers before questions have been completed
● Failure to wait in turn

- Interrupts or intrudes on others' conversations or games
- Talks constantly.

There must be some impairment in functioning both at home and at school. The symptoms cannot be accounted for by depression or anxiety.

The DSM definition of ADHD uses very similar criteria, but splits it into two groups instead of three: inattention and hyperactivity/impulsivity. The main reason that DSM-IV has a broader, more inclusive definition is that it requires *either* of these two symptom clusters rather than *all three* of the clusters, as in ICD-10.

Behaviour in the clinic is *not* a good indicator of the diagnosis. Most children with ADHD behave well for short periods of time (30–45 minutes) in a strange environment, particularly if provided with novel toys, or a supply of adult attention. In contrast, ***descriptions of behaviour in school*** by teachers *can* be a very good indicator of the diagnosis. Although parents who are good historians will give a reliable account of what the teacher has said to them, it is more reliable to get the information directly, preferably by sending questionnaires, either direct to the teacher or conveyed to school by parents. Rating scales can be useful, such as the Conners' in its earliest version, or more recent adaptations.[7] It is helpful in addition either to have a telephone conversation; or to set up a direct observation in school; or to send a more qualitative questionnaire, as shown in Box 31.3.

The problem of comorbidity

'Comorbidity' means the coexistence in one child of more than one disorder. This is common in ADHD, as already shown in Figure 31.1. ADHD may be associated with a variety of other developmental disorders. One particular combination of conditions is known as '***DAMP***' – Disorders of Attention, Motor Control and Perception.[8] These children have features of: ADHD; dyspraxia (the 'M' bit); and other specific learning difficulties or sensory impairments (the 'P' bit). A high proportion may have autistic features. This relatively recent term has taken over from the now outmoded term 'minimal brain dysfunction'. Another combination of conditions includes Tourette's disorder, ADHD and obsessive-compulsive symptoms (*see* Chapter 25 on Tics and Tourette's Syndrome): many such children also have oppositional defiant disorder (*see* Chapter 30) or at least significant behaviour problems.

The combination of ADHD with ***behaviour problems*** is *so* common, especially in boys, as to be quite confusing for many professionals, who view ADHD as almost synonymous with challenging behaviour. ADHD uncomplicated by behaviour problems can be seen in six- and seven-year-olds, often presenting as increasing impairment in the classroom. This presents an opportunity for the prevention of later behavioural problems by adequate treatment of the ADHD (*see* below). Untreated ADHD may lead to increasing dysfunction in the family, with friends and in school, contributing to the later development of delinquency, substance misuse and alienation from the education system. Many children known to Youth

BOX 31.3 Questionnaire for teachers

Name of child. . . . .   **Date:** . . . . / . . . . . /. . . . .
Name and role of teacher: . . . .

Academic progress:
estimated ability: below average / average / above average
school performance: underachieving / appropriate / over-striving

Special educational needs:
any difficulties with: reading / spelling / writing / language
any other educational difficulties?
what special provision is received (type of help; hours per week)?

Levels of activity and concentration:
attention span compared to other
children in class   better / the same / less / a lot less
distractibility   yes / no
repeatedly off seat or wandering around   yes / no
fidgeting   yes / no
ability to follow instructions   none at all / simple only / adequate
interrupts others   yes / no
tendency to do things without
thinking (impulsivity)   yes / no
organisational skills   above average / average / poor
frustration tolerance   above average / average / poor

Behaviour:
in the classroom
in the playground
at dinner time
Relationships with peers
Relationships with adults
Emotional development   anxiety / withdrawal / self-confidence / low self-esteem
Response to praise
Temperamental characteristics and adaptability
Parental involvement with the school
Any other comments

Offending Teams and in special schools for children with emotional and behavioural problems have ADHD, as do many adults in prison. *Impulsivity* leads to risk-taking: the child may have frequent accidents and be well known in his local Accident and Emergency department. ADHD makes adolescents more likely to start smoking early, experiment with sex but without contraception, or try drugs and alcohol. Part of this could be seen as self-medication for the ADHD symptoms – with nicotine in particular.

Children with ADHD can be *exhausting* to parent. Families may be reluctant to embark on any sort of outing, even to somewhere supposedly pleasurable and engrossing such as a theme park, for fear of it being so disrupted as to be unmanageable. Professionals should not underestimate the impact on family life of having a child with ADHD.

BOX 31.4 Practice Points for the assessment of ADHD

Does the child have difficulties in at least two of the three domains of home, school and friendships?

Does the child have enough of the three key features of ADHD to satisfy an ICD-10 diagnosis of hyperkinetic disorder?

If not, does the child have enough features of inattention or of hyperactivity/impulsivity to satisfy the DSM-IV criteria for ADHD?

Does the child have any specific or general learning difficulties?

Does the child have any other developmental problems?

Does the child have any of the other problems that may coexist with ADHD?

Does the child have any of the problems listed in Box 31.1 that may cause ADHD features (and may also coexist with ADHD)?

Is anything else happening at home or at school that may be causing the difficulties?

Does anyone else in the family have similar problems in childhood (even if not diagnosed)?

How are the rest of the family coping?

Is there any smoking or substance misuse in the family?

What measures have already been tried, at home or at school?

What is the family's view of the problem?

What are the child and parents hoping from professionals?

MANAGEMENT

Management consists of psychoeducation, behavioural approaches, medication and dietary advice.

Psychoeducation

Both the young person and others in his family need clear information, supplemented by appropriate resources, such as leaflets, booklets, videos, or information about support groups. It is important to explain the key features of ADHD and what this might make the young person do. The young person needs to be told that ADHD may make it more difficult for him to behave at times, especially when other people want him to sit still and complete tasks, but ADHD is not an excuse for bad behaviour. His tendency to fiddle, fidget and move in his seat should be ignored by parents and teachers: children with ADHD *can* concentrate if they are doing these things and this sort of movement may even *help* them concentrate. It may be worth a try to give a child with ADHD something to fiddle with, such as a squeezy ball or toy.

It is important to allow time to discuss the parents' or young person's beliefs and attitudes to ADHD and its management. In spite of increasing recognition of these problems, many incorrect beliefs and assumptions persist.

There is a variety of books and DVDs available; these are produced by charities, self-help groups, organisations concerned with mental health and the drug companies that manufacture the medications used in ADHD. The Internet is also a source of information: some is helpful and some misleading.

The role of medication and psychological approaches

Parents of children aged 3–8 years should ideally be offered parent training (group or individual) if the child has features of ADHD, whether or not a diagnosis of ADHD or oppositional defiant disorder has been confirmed. Medication should be reserved if possible for children of six years or over with severe ADHD, or children who are having significant problems in school that can be attributed to ADHD, and which have not responded to school-based interventions. Children may also benefit from group-based or individual psychological treatments such as cognitive-behavioural therapy or social skills training, if these are available.[9] The *behavioural management strategies* discussed below and how these are implemented will depend upon the age of the child, the severity of the ADHD symptoms and the parents' ability to make use of written information or other resources.

Inattention

Poor concentration and distractibility can be helped by environmental manipulation. This may mean providing a structure that helps the child cope with tasks more easily. Structure means the space around the child, the time he is expected to take, and the amount and frequency of adult attention he receives. Attention should be positive or rewarding as much as possible (for instance, joining in with the play activity, or praising any small achievement).

➤ Provide an environment in which there is a minimum of distraction, at least for parts of the day (for instance, a small room with few objects, or a table facing the corner of the classroom). To make this work, there need to be predictable times when social contact occurs (with teacher, non-teaching assistant or other children). This principle can be applied at home to help with particular tasks, such as homework or creative play.

➤ Break tasks down into the smallest possible components. For instance ,a sheet of homework with 10 questions on it may be broken down into two lots of four and one of two so that the child can be helped to complete it in these three chunks, with short gaps between to move around or attend to any pressing distractions. Make sure that all tasks set are achievable, by adjusting the standard to the child – for instance, for the amount and accuracy of work, or the amount of mess allowed.

➤ Provide a suitable time frame. It is unrealistic to expect a child with ADHD to stick at one task for a long period. Allow brief spells at the task, with frequent breaks.

➤ Reward each task or sub-task when completed, half completed or attempted, at every opportunity – usually with labelled praise (*see* Chapter 13 on Behaviour Management and general behaviour and compliance below).

➤ Try to build up the duration of concentration gradually, step by step.

➤ If continual adult attention cannot be provided, try to find stimulating activities which the child can do on his own or with other children.

➤ Cards or posters with lists of rules and goals may be useful. They can be put on the wall of the child's room at home, or on his desk at school. Cards can be used to prompt desired behaviours, such as tidying up, and provide a time frame, such as for five minutes after homework or playing.

Impulsivity

A lack of inhibition may be a central problem in ADHD. It is also one of the most difficult aspects to manage, but some of the strategies below may help. It can be a challenge to teach greater social awareness and problem-solving, so think of ways of keeping the child on task, such as frequent rewards and doing no more than a little bit at a time. (There is more on problem-solving in Chapter 13.)

➤ Encourage the child to talk about his thoughts and plans and strategies for doing things. For instance, if he is good at computer games, get him to talk through what exactly he does. Then try talking through what happened recently in the playground, or with a sibling or a friend at home.

➤ Define a problem (for instance: getting into fights in the playground, getting frustrated when the computer game doesn't go right, not being able to do more than five minutes homework a night).

➤ Encourage him to think how this made him feel.

➤ Encourage him to think how this made the other person or people in the situation feel.

➤ Think with him about the reasons for feelings, and how one event may lead to another over time.

➤ Brainstorm a number of alternative solutions. Some of these may be daft – don't rule out any solutions yet. Together, you could note down good and daft ideas on paper, or on a computer. This is easier to do if it is in concrete form, but once he has got used to the process, you can forget the paper or the computer, and do it just by talking, and then eventually he can do it on his own just by thinking. For instance, you could have a rule of thumb to think of three alternatives, and then decide which one seems best.

➤ Discuss each possible solution, and think about how it might make things different, or what the consequences might be.

➤ Choose one of the possible solutions, and make a plan based on this for what he will do next time the situation arises.

➤ Rehearse it.

➤ Encourage him to think before he acts next time the problem situation arises – at any rate for long enough to apply the new solution (easier said than done).

➤ Make sure to check if he has carried this plan out. If he hasn't, go on encouraging him until he does. If he has, go through it with him as soon as possible afterwards to review how he has succeeded. You may need to go through the problem-solving process several times to find a really successful strategy.

General behaviour and compliance

Techniques for behavioural management are the same as for other children of the same age, but the ADHD may make it rather more of a challenge to achieve success with these techniques.

➤ List the child's positive attributes.

➤ What would you like him to be able to achieve?

➤ Think of the difficulties that his condition makes for him. Think how much more he is achieving than other children without ADHD when he completes even a simple task.

➤ Think about how negatively he makes you feel.

➤ Think how poorly he must view himself.

➤ Try to help him feel better about himself whenever possible. Praise should be frequent, reinforced by eye contact and other non-verbal cues, and labelled. For instance, 'I really like that drawing of a car you've done – it looks so powerful!', or 'Thank you for tidying up straight away after you finished that game' [hug]. Labelled praise should be the main reward.

➤ Make all praise and rewards immediate.

➤ If you use tangible rewards, such as points systems or presents, vary them frequently.

➤ Try to find opportunities for doing things together you both enjoy. Ten minutes a day playing together is enough to make a difference, although it can seem very hard to find this time.

➤ When giving commands, gain the child's attention by making eye contact and persuading him to stop what he is doing and listen. Make requests simple and specific, so that he knows exactly what he has to do. It may help to get him to repeat what you have asked him to do. Avoid sequences of commands, vague commands or giving several commands at once. Wait 10 seconds for him to comply – praise him immediately when he does.

➤ If he does not comply, remember it does not help to blame this on yourself or on him – blame the ADHD.

➤ Using more punishments than rewards may make things worse.

➤ Coordination between strategies at home and school makes both more effective.

➤ Set up routines for certain behaviours on certain days. For instance, a sequence of activities is needed for getting up and going to school, and different ones for the weekend. Prompt cards may help with these.

See also Chapter 13 on Behaviour Management.

Hyperactivity

Children with ADHD are restless, get up and down, like to move and fidget, fiddle with things and may be poorly co-ordinated. They find it hard to reduce this motor activity. Attempts to get them to stop fiddling, fidgeting, rocking or moving are usually unproductive.

➤ Therefore it is best to ignore fiddling, fidgeting or squirming.

➤ Try giving the child something innocuous to fiddle with.

➤ Strongly encourage any opportunity for physical activity or sport, for instance in lunchtime, after-school or weekend clubs.

➤ In the classroom, it may help to let a child with ADHD get up and down to pass things around or to collect things up, or take messages (or the register) to the office. He is more likely to do this than to sit still in his seat whilst someone else does it.

➤ At school, keeping him in at playtime as a punishment is likely to make things worse, as he probably needs to get out of the classroom and run around.

➤ Similarly at home, it is best to allow the child to be hyperactive whenever possible, rather than trying to restrain him or ground him. For instance, getting up at mealtimes or climbing all over the furniture has to be tolerated.

Medication

Medication is recommended only for the most severe ADHD with marked impairment of function, particularly at school.[10] For children over six years of age with significant symptoms at school, stimulant medication may be the most effective initial treatment. The only *stimulant medications* available in the UK are methylphenidate and dexamfetamine. Methylphenidate is available in a variety of preparations of different duration (*see* Figure 31.3). Dexamfetamine is available in only one preparation (Dexedrine) and only in short-acting form. The main *non-stimulant* is atomoxetine (Strattera), which unfortunately has just as many side effects (perhaps more). It may be useful when symptoms at home are more of a concern than symptoms at school (in which case some form of behavioural treatment should be tried first if available).

Medication should be started only after a specialist who is an expert in ADHD (usually a paediatrician or child psychiatrist) has thoroughly assessed the child or adolescent and established the diagnosis. Once treatment has been started it can be continued and monitored by a general practitioner. Medication should be

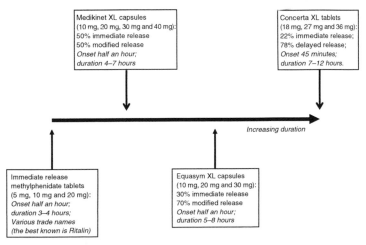

FIGURE 31.3 Duration of action of different preparations of methylphenidate

monitored regularly, usually by both the specialist and the general practitioner under a shared care protocol.

For the core symptoms of ADHD, medication is effective in about 70% of cases. Stimulants are effective rapidly, from the first day they are taken. They have a direct effect on attention, short-term memory, vigilance, reaction time, listening skills and on-task behaviour. Side-effects include appetite suppression (which can lead to weight loss and sometimes reduced height velocity and therefore final height), delayed sleep onset, increased emotionality or obsessionality, headaches, tummy aches, nausea, excessive calmness and worsening of pre-existing tics.

Children with ADHD who are taking stimulant medication are likely to feel different and experience negative attitudes from peers, teachers and the public – which they attribute to the diagnosis of ADHD and the disruptive behaviour it causes more than their medication.[11] They commonly experience bullying, but attribute this more to their ADHD behaviours than the need to take medication. They credit the medication with improving their social behaviour and relationships.

Atomoxetine (Strattera) works more on overall calmness than concentration, and has a slight anti-anxiety effect. It may take up to six weeks before the effect is established, and the medication has to be taken once every day (in the mornings or evenings). When the effect has built up, it works 24 hours a day, which may be beneficial for family functioning. Side effects include appetite suppression, drowsiness, headaches, nausea, vomiting, dizziness and suicidal ideas.

Dietary intervention

All children will benefit from a balanced diet and regular exercise. There is plentiful evidence that *dietary exclusion* can improve the behaviour of many children but it is less clear whether this can be seen as a treatment specifically for ADHD.[12,13,14] It is worth asking whether carers have noticed any foods or drinks worsening the child's behaviour or leading to hyperactivity. A food diary with comments about behaviour may help, but unfortunately parental observation is significantly affected by parental expectation.[15] Exclusion of culprit foods should be cautiously encouraged, but if this shows any likelihood of leading to excessive dietary restriction or an inadequate diet, then a paediatric dietician should be involved.[16,17]

Some parents choose to try *dietary supplementation*, for instance with omega-3 fatty acids (fish oils). There is conflicting evidence as to whether this works for all or more likely *some* of the symptoms of ADHD (*see* Chapter 44 on Diet and Exercise): at the time of writing this chapter, there have been five studies showing omega-3 supplementation to be effective and five showing it to be ineffective.[18] So it is not yet sufficiently evidence-based to justify the National Health Service paying for prescriptions of these supplements. Some parents are prepared to pay fully for them, for instance out of the child's Disability Living Allowance. Given that there seem to be overall health benefits from omega-3 supplementation, and no evidence that the present authors are aware of indicating harm, this could be cautiously encouraged, providing it does not lead to financial hardship.

BOX 31.5 Case Example

Harry is a six-year-old boy in his second year of primary school. His mother, Clare, is concerned because he doesn't seem to be keeping up with work in class, and whenever she picks him up at school, the teacher tells her about a different sort of trouble he has got into. Although Harry has had friends home to play, they don't seem to come back a second time. He seems to be very accident-prone, always falling over, bruising and cutting himself. Harry and Clare and his two-year-old half-sister, Joely, live with Joely's father next to a park, so Harry can play there while Clare keeps an eye on him from the house. Inside, he is always getting in everyone else's way and interrupting things.

The head teacher asks the social inclusion pupil support worker to become involved, which Clare finds a bit concerning. Fortunately, they get on well. The social inclusion pupil support worker points out that Harry has difficulty concentrating in class, as well as being hyperactive. After discussing Harry's behaviour, they realise he is also impulsive. The social inclusion pupil support worker discusses with Harry's class teacher how he can be helped in class, for instance by sitting close to the front at a corner of the classroom, and being allowed breaks between tasks. Harry is also discussed in the next consultation meeting with the school's educational psychologist, who suggests further measures that might help Harry achieve more in lessons, such as breaking down his schoolwork into manageable bits, and to some extent differentiating his work from the rest of the class. Harry's class teacher says she is concerned that Harry is not making enough progress with literacy skills, so the educational psychologist agrees to arrange some relevant testing.

The social inclusion pupil support worker is able to find a behaviour management course for Clare to go on, although Clare is a bit reluctant, as she sees the main problem as being in school: she has found ways of coping at home. Clare goes on the course, on condition that she can also have a referral to the local community paediatrician, who runs an ADHD clinic. By the time Harry gets to the paediatric ADHD clinic, Clare has completed the parenting course, which she has found more helpful than she expected. The results of the specific literacy tests are back, showing that Harry is about 18 months behind his chronological age in reading, spelling and writing skills. Once the community paediatrician has received a report from the school, she has little hesitation in diagnosing ADHD. Clare decides that medication may help Harry in class so would be worth a try.

Harry starts on short-acting methylphenidate, and after gradually building up the dose, seems to do best on 10 mg at breakfast-time and 5 mg at lunchtime. He is a lot better in the mornings but still hyperactive and easily distractible in the afternoons. However, a 10 mg lunchtime dose seems to keep him awake until midnight, whereas with 5 mg he gets to sleep between 9 and 10 pm.

Three years later, Harry has caught up in his reading and spelling attainments, although he is still six months behind his chronological age and continues to have extra support with literacy. His parents still find him hyperactive at home in the evenings and before he goes to school, but are pleased that he is enjoying school and able to bring a couple of best friends home repeatedly. Harry attends three after-school clubs on weekday evenings and trains with his football club on Saturdays. He mostly tolerates his sister Joely. He is now on long-acting Equasym XL 40 mg on school days and Saturdays, Ritalin 10 mg after school on days when he has clubs, and melatonin 10 mg at night, without which it is difficult for him to get off to sleep.

LONG-TERM OUTCOME

The long-term prognosis for children and adolescents with ADHD is highly variable and depends on a number of factors. Although hyperactivity tends to subside in adolescence, most other ADHD symptoms – particularly disorganisation and inattention – can persist into adulthood and cause significant impairment, for instance in occupational achievement, relationship stability or criminality. Management is complicated by comorbidity, for instance with antisocial personality disorder. Adequate transitional arrangements for transfer of care to adult mental health services may be hard to achieve in some areas.

REFERRAL

The pathway for referral of ADHD varies geographically, but should ideally involve local educational psychologists, paediatricians and child psychiatrists in specialist assessment.

RESOURCES
Websites

- ADDNet UK has a useful website, with links to others, at: www.web-tv.co.uk
- ADDISS is the main UK parent support organisation at present: www.addiss.co.uk

Books for parents

- Dendy CAZ. *Teenagers with ADD and ADHD: a guide for parents and professionals.* Bethesda, MD: Woodbine House; 2005.
  This North American guide to understanding and coping with teenagers who have ADHD discusses diagnosis, medical treatment, family and school life, interventions, advocacy, legal rights and options after school.
- Laver-Bradbury C, Thompson M, Weeks A, *et al. Step by Step Help for Children with ADHD: a self-help manual for parents.* London: Jessica Kingsley; 2011.
  Written by an experienced team from Southampton, this practical guide describes their flexible six-step programme and includes techniques and strategies that parents can practice, ideas for developing communication with the child's school, games that will help improve the child s attention, exercises to develop patience and tips for supporting the child in successful self-organization.
- Mental Health Foundation. *All about ADHD.* London: Mental Health Foundation; 2000.
  A small booklet giving convenient basic information, available for £1 from: The Mental Health Foundation, 20/21, Cornwall Terrace, London NW1 4QL; telephone 020 7535 7400; fax 020 7535 7474; e-mail mhf@mhf.org.uk or at the www.mhf.org.uk website.
- Parker HC. *Put Yourself in Their Shoes: understanding teenagers with attention deficit hyperactivity disorder.* Michigan: Partners Publishing Group; 1999.
  This is for anyone who wants practical information on how to help a teenager with ADHD and covers topics such as: family communication, promoting responsibility, study strategies, college and vocational training, and more.
- Pentecost D. *Parenting the ADD Child: Can't do? Won't do? Practical strategies for managing behaviour problems in children with ADD and ADHD.* London: Jessica Kingsley Publications; 2000.

Each chapter has practical strategies for dealing with a child with ADHD.

- Taylor E. *Understanding your Hyperactive Child: the essential guide for parents.* London: Vermilion; 1997.
  A book full of information by the leading British authority on the subject.

Books for children

- Chilman-Blair K, Taddeo J, Hill PD. *What's Up With Astra? Medikidz explain ADHD.* London: Medikidz Foundation; 2010.
  One in a series of UK books in graphic novel format explaining childhood disorders to children, this volume explores the different lobes of the brain and introduces the chemical messengers Nora and Dopey.
- Corman CL, Trevino E, DiMatteo RA. *Eukee the Jumpy Jumpy Elephant.* Minnesota: Specialty Press; 2010.
  This story for children aged four to eight years describes a hyperactive elephant who moves through the jungle like a tornado, unable to pay attention like the other elephants. He begins to feel sad, but gets help after a visit to the doctor.
- Moss DM, Schwartz C. *Shelley, the Hyperactive Turtle.* Bethesda, MD: Woodbine House; 2006.
  This story for children aged four to eight years describes a bright young turtle who is not like other turtles.
- Nadeau KG, Dixon EB, Beyl C. *Learning to Slow Down and Pay Attention: a book for kids about ADHD.* 3rd ed. Washington DC: Magination Press (American Psychological Association); 2004.
  This book is aimed at children aged eight to 12 years, and uses fun cartoons, games, activities and graphics to give children a variety of coping strategies.
- Quinn PO, Stern JM, Lee J. *Putting on the Brakes: Understanding and taking control of your ADD or ADHD.* 2nd ed. Washington DC: Magination Press (American Psychological Association); 2009.
  This book for children of nine to 12 years focuses on the feelings and emotions of children with ADHD and suggests specific techniques for gaining control of the situation, becoming better organised, and functioning better at school, home and with friends.
- Quinn PO, Stern JM, Lee J. *Putting on the Brakes Activity Book for Kids with ADD or ADHD.* Washington DC: Magination Press (American Psychological Association); 2009.
  This activity book is a companion to the above and allows children to put their understanding of ADHD into action.
- Wever C, Phillips N. *Full of Beans.* New South Wales: Shrink-Rap Press (Australia) Pty Ltd; 2007.
  This splendid creation explains all he needs to know about ADHD to any child who likes looking at pictures or reading. www.shrinkrap.com.au/fullofbeans.html

REFERENCES

1 Sayal K. Epidemiology of attention-deficit/hyperactivity disorder in the community. *British Journal of Hospital Medicine.* 2007; **68**(7): 352–5.
2 National Institute for Health and Clinical Excellence. *Attention Deficit Hyperactivity Disorder: diagnosis and management of ADHD in children, young people and adults* [clinical guideline CG72]. London: National Institute for Health and Clinical Excellence; 2008. Available at: http://guidance.nice.org.uk/CG72 (accessed 2 April 2011).

3 Williams R, Richardson G, Kurtz Z, *et al.* The definition, epidemiology and nature of child and adolescent mental health problems and disorders. In: Health Advisory Service, editor. *Child and Adolescent Mental Health Services: together we stand.* London: HMSO; 1995. pp. 15–25.

4 World Health Organisation. *The ICD-10 Classification of Mental and Behavioural Disorders: diagnostic criteria for research.* Geneva: World Health Organization; 1993.

5 American Psychiatric Association. *Diagnostic and Statistical Manual of Mental Disorders.* Washington, DC: American Psychiatric Association; 1994.

6 National Institute for Health and Clinical Excellence, op. cit.

7 Conners K. Rating scales for use in drug studies with children. *Psychopharmacology Bulletin: special issue on pharmacotherapy with children.* 1973; **9**: 24–84.

8 Gillberg C. Deficits in attention, motor control and perception: a brief review. *Arch Dis Child.* 2003; **88**(10): 904–10.

9 National Institute for Health and Clinical Excellence, op. cit.

10 National Institute for Health and Clinical Excellence, op. cit.

11 Singh I, Kendall T, Taylor C, *et al.* Young people's experience of ADHD and stimulant medication: a qualitative study for the NICE Guideline. *Child and Adolescent Mental Health.* 2010; **15**(4): 186–92.

12 McCann D, Barrett A, Cooper A, *et al.* Food additives and hyperactive behaviour in 3-year-old and 8/9-year-old children in the community: a randomised, double-blinded, placebo-controlled trial. *Lancet.* 2007 Nov 3; **370**: 1560–7.

13 Bateman B, Warner JO, Hutchinson E, *et al.* The effects of a double blind, placebo controlled, artificial food colourings and benzoate preservative challenge on hyperactivity in a general population sample of preschool children. *Arch Dis Child.* 2004; **89**(6): 506–11.

14 Schab DW, Trinh NH. Do artificial food colors promote hyperactivity in children with hyperactive syndromes? A meta-analysis of double-blind placebo-controlled trials. *J Dev Behav Pediatr.* 2004; **25**(6): 423–34.

15 Bateman, op. cit.

16 Kemp A. Food additives and hyperactivity. *BMJ.* 2008; **336**(7654): 1144.

17 National Institute for Health and Clinical Excellence, op. cit.

18 Richardson AJ. Omega-3 for behaviour, learning and mood: what's the real evidence? Presentation given at Food and Behaviour Research Conference, *Feeding Success: why better nutrition is vital for improving mental health and performance.* 2010 Sep 23. Saïd Business School, Oxford.

CHAPTER 32

Developmental disorders, Part 2: Autistic spectrum disorders

INTRODUCTION

Epidemiology

Recently, the phrase *'autism epidemic'* has been used to describe the steadily increasing numbers of people recognized as having autism or at least an autistic spectrum disorder. It remains a matter of debate as to whether this is due to a combination of increased awareness and a progressive relaxation of the thresholds for diagnosis, or alternatively to a genuine increase in prevalence (due to factors unknown – but certainly not immunisations). An intriguing hypothesis is that our (Western) civilisation has increasingly emphasised left hemisphere functions in preference to right, which makes us all more autistic, because autism is characterised by a lack of right-hemisphere functions and an exaggerated reliance on the left: so the increase in prevalence at the impairment end of the autistic spectrum is real.[1]

Historically, the prevalence of 'typical' or 'core' autism was said to be about 2–5 per 10,000 of the population – the majority of such cases also have learning disability.[2] Over the past decade or more there has been a shift from a tight categorical view of autism to a dimensional understanding, leading to an increasingly inclusive diagnostic sieve.[3] The shift to diagnoses on the spectrum instead of at the core has led to prevalence rates of the order of 1%.[4,5,6] In practice, this means that anyone working with a number of children at the Tier 1 and 2 levels is likely to encounter many children with autistic features, and probably some with an autistic spectrum disorder.

Terminology

Autistic spectrum disorder (or autism spectrum disorder or autistic spectrum condition) are inclusive terms that cover a variety of previously separated conditions. They are roughly equivalent to the ICD-10 term 'pervasive developmental disorder' and include for instance: autism, high-functioning autism, Asperger's disorder, atypical autism, and pervasive developmental disorder not otherwise specified.[7]

The underlying problem is generally agreed to be atypical neurodevelopment. Because not all affected individuals show impairment, some prefer the word 'condition' to the word 'disorder'. Those who prefer the term 'autism spectrum' to 'autistic spectrum' argue that it is not the spectrum that is autistic, but the children (we contend that the same misplaced argument could be used about the phrase 'electromagnetic spectrum'). The term 'spectrum' is used because, while all people with an autistic diagnosis should to some extent have difficulties in the three main areas (*see* next paragraph), their condition may affect them in very different ways. Many are able to live functional everyday lives; at the other extreme, some will require a lifetime of specialist support.

SUMMARY OF FEATURES

People with an autistic spectrum disorder have difficulty in three main areas which are known as the ***triad of impairments***. They are:
➤ difficulty with social communication
➤ difficulty with social interaction
➤ repetitive behaviours, restricted interests and difficulty with change.

Associated features that are not essential for a diagnosis but may be part of the overall picture include the following:
➤ some form of sensory sensitivity
➤ some form of motor incoordination
➤ a generalised learning disability
➤ special abilities, commonly musical, mathematical, or in visualisation (a particular skill in drawing or architecture) – these special abilities have been denoted by the phrase 'idiot savant'
➤ a specific learning disability or a combination of skills in some areas with deficits in others
➤ other developmental disorders such as ADHD or Tourette's disorder
➤ other psychiatric disorders such as obsessive compulsive-disorder or depression
➤ psychotic symptoms that are qualitatively differ from those seen in psychotic illness (*see* Chapter 45 on Imaginary Friends, Voices and Psychosis)
➤ neurological disorders such as epilepsy
➤ gastrointestinal problems such as irritable bowel syndrome or food intolerances
➤ genetic syndromes such as Fragile X or tuberous sclerosis.

Autistic spectrum disorders are more common in boys than girls, though may be under-diagnosed in girls, because they present differently. A relevant analysis from the Avon Longitudinal Study suggest that the ratio of boys to girls may be about 7:1.[8]

BOX 32.1 Case Example

Edmund is a 17-year-old boy who is fascinated by bodybuilding and has a large collection of magazines showing muscular physiques. He takes lots of exercise, and eats mainly protein. He had difficulties at school, where he was thought to have Asperger's disorder without learning difficulties, but has now left school, and will not go to college or socialise with friends. He reluctantly admits that he has started vomiting. His mother is very concerned at how much weight he has lost in the last three months.

Assessment by Tier 3 CAMHS suggests that the underlying problem is Asperger's disorder, but the acute problem that needs treating is anorexia nervosa. After a period of compulsory admission to a medical ward to stabilise Edmund's physiology, he reluctantly revises his dietary habits and stops himself vomiting in order to avoid admission to psychiatric hospital. Follow-up at increasing intervals shows that Edmund's diet, although very solitary and obsessional, is now sufficient for him to gain weight, which he continues to do until discharge from the CAMHS service at the age of 18½ years.

The involved professionals view Edmund's Asperger's disorder as not only having led to his eating disorder, perhaps via mechanisms including obsessionality and sensory sensitivity, but also having given him a way of overcoming it.

BOX 32.2 Case Example

Solomon is 14 years old when his Head of Year mentions to the community school nurse that some of his teachers think he may have Asperger's disorder. He is very good at mathematics and computing, but does not work well in groups. He can get on very well with some of his subject teachers but clashes with others. He does not seem to have any close friends. The community school nurse asks whether these concerns have been discussed with his parents. The Head of Year says she tried to broach the issue with both Solomon's parents at a parents' evening, but they were very dismissive. She offered them the opportunity to meet with her for a more private discussion, but they did not telephone to arrange an appointment.

The community school nurse telephones Solomon's mother to explain that she would like to meet with both parents to discuss something the school is concerned about that she can't easily discuss over the telephone. Solomon's mother pauses, then says it would be all right for the nurse to visit during a day when she is not working but Solomon's father is.

At the home visit, Solomon's mother says that she is aware of the school's concern that Solomon may have Asperger's disorder, but his father is very much against the use of labels. He doesn't think there is anything much wrong with Solomon, and remembers being very similar when he himself was at school. Solomon's mother asks the community school nurse what difference a diagnosis might make, if she could persuade his father to allow him to be assessed. The community school nurse says she is not sure, and they don't even know whether Solomon has enough features to merit a diagnosis, but if he did, this might perhaps lead to some extra support in school and subsequently at college or university. A diagnosis might also enable Solomon to understand his own difficulties better (for instance with friends) and choose the sort of job that would make demands on his strengths rather than his weaknesses.

They agree that Solomon's parents will discuss things and get back to the nurse if they want to take things further; she agrees not to say anything at all to Solomon. After a month, the community school nurse has heard nothing, so she telephones Solomon's mother to ask what she has decided. Solomon's mother explains that his father does not think it would be helpful to have professionals prying into their family, and he thinks Solomon is doing quite well enough at school not to need any further help. The nurse asks whether she can say anything to the Head of Year; after thinking a bit, Solomon's mother says the nurse can tell the Head of Year that his parents have discussed things and are aware of the school's concerns and grateful for their support, but do not want to take things any further at present.

BOX 32.3 Autism and Asperger's syndrome – key features and main differences

Both have:
- difficulties with social communication and interaction
- fixated interests and repetitive behaviours.

The main differences are slight, and more degree than substance.
- The relevant differences are by definition noted at an earlier age in autism.
- The intelligence quotient tends to be average or above-average in Asperger's syndrome, but can be any level in autism.
- The level of overall disability is generally milder in Asperger's (but the situation can vary with time and maturation).

DETAILS OF THE MAIN FEATURES

These vary from one person to another but can be divided into the three main areas described above as the *triad of impairments*. In any one child on the autistic spectrum, some skills may be deficient while others are intact (or greater than average): during assessment, it is important to build up an overall picture of strengths and weaknesses.

Social communication

An individual on the autistic spectrum tends to have *difficulties with social communication* – both *verbal and non-verbal*. The level of verbal language varies greatly – some young people with autism may use very few if any words; if so, it is often difficult to assess the intelligence quotient. Such an autist may nevertheless understand what other people say to him. Whether he does or not, he may prefer to use alternative means of communication such as a form of sign language, or visual symbols such as the Picture Exchange Communication System (PECS).[9] Other autistic individuals may have good language skills, superficially within the normal range, but nevertheless a literal understanding of language combined with a lack of appreciation of the influence of context on meaning that handicaps their social interaction. Difficulties may arise, for example, with common phrases or sayings such as: 'Pull your socks up!' or 'Get a move on!' as well as sarcasm and other jokes. Even as innocent-sounding a phrase as 'Wait a minute …' may lead to frustration or fury when the adult takes longer than a minute (*see also* Case Example in Box 32.18 below).

BOX 32.4 Case Example

> Gareth, aged nine years, has high-functioning autism. He is good at lessons but finds unstructured times difficult, particularly lunch breaks. He clashes with a dinner lady who perceives him as naughty. She tells him to 'get a move on and sit down to have your lunch!' He perceives these two instructions as contradictory, and is unable to respond to either command, leading to *his* increasing distress and confirmation from *her* point of view that he is disobedient.

Some children speak in an overly formal way, perhaps sounding like a mini-professor, using adult-type language or repeating phrases and words they have heard without really understanding their meaning. Such a child's **speech** may sound formal or monotonous or lack inflection and variation. He may find it hard to understand the give-and-take nature of conversations, perhaps repeating what the other person has just said (echolalia) or talking at length about his own interests regardless of how the other person responds or whether she shows any interest.

Non-verbal communication difficulties may occur, such as infrequent eye contact or smiling, inappropriate gestures, problems with turn-taking or misinterpretations of others' facial expressions, tone of voice or gestures. Such a child may fail to respond appropriately to another's distress, for instance not knowing what to do when someone cries or shows disappointment. He may therefore be perceived as being rude, not helped by a lack of tact; he may announce at full volume while on the bus: 'Look at that fat lady over there, mummy!'

Social interaction

All of this contributes to *difficulties with social interaction*. A child on the autistic spectrum often has difficulty with the *recognition of emotion*. There are two elements to this: one is the recognition and labelling of one's own emotions, in which an autistic child is likely to be deficient; the other is recognising those same emotions in others (part of a theory of mind). This can make it difficult for him to fit in socially. He may not tune in to the unwritten social rules that most of us intuit without necessarily thinking about them. Examples of social gaucheness may include:

➤ standing too close to another person – invading personal space – this may be due to poor kinaesthetic sensation (bodily awareness) rather than poor social understanding – *see* below

> changing the subject of conversation inappropriately
> talking about something inappropriate or irrelevant to some or all of the listeners
> not recognising how someone is feeling and therefore reacting awkwardly
> behaving in ways that are perceived by others as strange or eccentric
> preferring to spend time alone rather than with others.

BOX 32.5 Case Example

In her two final years of secondary school, Lucy feels unable to attend. She has difficulty explaining what makes school difficult for her, but it seems she cannot get on with her teachers or other pupils. Her parents find her quite exasperating, as she will not participate in any conversation about solutions for her education, refuses to join in family activities and yet encroaches on their personal space. Nevertheless, once given a place at college, Lucy not only attends but manages to fit in, finding a course that suits her and a boyfriend who dotes on her.

The girl described in Box 32.5 never gets a formal diagnosis, but her underlying difficulties could be seen as autistic in nature: social situations leading to anxiety leading to avoidance of school, lack of age-appropriate ability to discuss feelings and solutions, inability to respect another's need for personal space.

All of the above make it difficult to form or sustain *friendships*. Some autistic children would like to make friends more successfully, and are frustrated that they don't; others seem to prefer to be alone, being apparently uninterested in seeking friendship. The combination of oddness and social isolation makes an autistic child a ready victim of bullying, but his response may vary. A few children may be able to ignore taunts and teasing, in which case these are likely to fade away. More commonly, a child on the autistic spectrum may experience any minor adverse comment as an episode of bullying, and then either complain about it vociferously to the surrounding school staff, who do not perceive any significant bullying – or more likely overreact with aggression so that the situation tends to escalate, and he is the one who gets into trouble.

Social imagination encompasses skills such as the following:
> Understanding the intent or meaning of other people's behaviour
> Interpreting what is behind the behaviour of others – thoughts, feelings or wishes
> Predicting the future behaviour of others. A concrete example involves anticipating the course of traffic, so not running onto a busy road. A more abstract example involves anticipating a parent's response to a distressed baby
> Imagining situations outside of everyday experience. Autistic children may enjoy imaginative play, but usually prefer to act out the same scenes each time. This means that joint imaginative play with other children will proceed smoothly only if it follows the autistic child's agenda. Imagination itself (as opposed to social imagination) may be heightened in areas of high ability, such as music, drawing, painting, acting or writing

➤ Coping in new or unfamiliar situations
➤ Planning for the future – if it differs significantly from the present
➤ Comprehending abstract ideas of the sort that many adolescents enjoy getting their heads round. Examples include: group decision-making processes such as democracy, moral viewpoints such as altruism or empathy, and the tug-of-war between dependence and independence.

Difficulties with such components of social imagination mean a young person on the autistic spectrum may in various ways be on the periphery of the social world around him.

BOX 32.6 Case Example

> Harish, aged seven years, has friends home from school – invited by his parents – but they tend not to visit more than once. His mother notices that Harish decides exactly what to do, and if the visitor wants to do something else, Harish lets him get on with it and merely plays on his own.

Repetitive behaviours, restricted interests and difficulty with change
The third area of difficulty is an amalgam of various core autistic features not included in the other two areas.

A young person on the autistic spectrum tends to like **routines**, sameness and predictability. A routine is something that has to be done at the same time every day. This repeated activity may grow into a **ritual** if it consists of a sequence of activities that have to be repeated in the same order on every occasion, sometimes including repetition of one or more components a certain number of times; often it has to be repeated from the beginning if interrupted or done incorrectly. In more extreme degrees of autism, repetitive behaviours may take the form of hand-flapping, rocking, spinning or other stereotyped movements.

Some rituals may be very elaborate and time consuming, so can come to dominate family life. This sort of symptom overlaps with obsessive-compulsive disorder, but there can be differences in the nature of the compulsions: for instance, rituals in obsessive-compulsive disorder are often based on a need for cleanliness or concerns about disease, whereas in autistic spectrum disorder, it may be harder to see meaning in the nature of the repeated behaviours.[10]

BOX 32.7 Case Example

> Matthew, aged 12 years, has a morning routine that makes it difficult for him to get to school on time. He has to tie both his shoelaces into a double bow with the ends exactly the same length, and there are only two pairs of trousers he will agree to wear. He has to have two Weetabix with the milk poured around them, not on top, so that only he can do this properly. His orange juice has to be in the same beaker every morning, filled up to exactly two-thirds full.

The world can seem a very unpredictable and confusing place to a young person on the autistic spectrum. It can be made more predictable and less confusing by having a fixed daily routine – to get as close as possible to a situation in which he knows what is going to happen each day and when. Examples of such comforting routines include travelling the same way to and from school; or eating exactly the same food in the same order for breakfast every day. If the established routine is interrupted, the young person may become extremely anxious. Sometimes this *anxiety* may erupt in the form of an aggressive or destructive outburst. A child on the autistic spectrum may find it extremely difficult to cope with simple changes of routine that most would take in their stride. Examples include: having a supply teacher unexpectedly replace the regular class teacher, having plans for a weekend activity suddenly changed, or coping with an unusual school day timetable (sports day, the week before Christmas or school trips). Such a child can usually cope better if he is prepared for the change in advance and given as much warning as possible. Introducing visual schedules or timetables can be extremely helpful (*see* below).

Rules may also be important to a young person on the autistic spectrum, in several different ways. Examples include the following.

➤ It may be difficult for him to take a different approach to something once he has been taught the 'right' way to do it.

➤ If he is punished in a certain way for breaking a particular rule, then he may find it difficult to accept that another child gets a different consequence for breaking the same rule.

➤ If a certain consequence for rule-infringement is promised, then nothing happens, the young person may view the adult (teacher or parent) as a liar (and lying is of course wrong).

➤ He may remember examples of (perceived) unfairness for a long time. This may at times lead to retaliation, which may occasionally be of a dangerous nature.

BOX 32.8 Case Example

> Patrick, aged nine years, is a pupil at a special school for moderated learning difficulties. Unbeknown to his teachers, he forms the idea that another pupil has not been adequately punished for saying something rude to him. A few days after a particular episode that upset him, Patrick somehow gets to be alone with the other pupil when all the others have left the classroom. He manages to barricade the door with some of the chairs, and uses another chair to smash over the other pupil's head.
>
> When questioned afterwards, Patrick can only say that the other boy deserved what happened to him; he seems unable to acknowledge the social inappropriateness, the disproportionality or the harmful consequences of what he has done.

Interests tend to be narrow and obsessional in nature. A young person on the autistic spectrum is likely to have intense special interests, often from a young age, that in general are not shared with others. These may change over time or be lifelong, and can take almost any form. Some interests may lead to a choice of career that fits with the interest, such as: music, drawing, computers, animals, trains or sports results. Others may remain solely a hobby. Some interests may appear initially to be peer-related, such as Dr Who, Pokémon, Yu-Gi-Oh cards, Warhammer or console games, but diverge in time from the interests of peers in pattern and degree. Examples of odd or bizarre interests include barcodes, grids, fire extinguishers or pylons.

Interests are likely to be:

➤ solitary rather than shared – exclusive of other people
➤ exclusive of other activities
➤ persistent rather than fleeting
➤ dominant in the household, overriding others' needs.

Some children develop an obsession with imaginary friends or worlds, but this is not necessarily an autistic characteristic (*see* Chapter 45 on Imaginary friends, voices and psychosis). Girls on the autistic spectrum may have different special interests from boys, such as animals, toy figures, television characters or make-up, making them less obviously different from their peers.

BOX 32.9 Case Example

Jane, a 10-year-old girl with Asperger's syndrome, loves her Go-Go's (small plastic figures). She has a large number of these and has created her own world with her collection in a part of her room. She can spend hours playing with them on her own in a repetitive way. She is seen as odd by her classmates, none of whom currently share this interest.

BOX 32.10 Case Example

Clare is a teenage girl who has always struggled with social relationships and feels different from her peers. She loves baking cakes: she takes a photo of every cake that she bakes (not just those for special occasions) and has to keep all these photos.

BOX 32.11 Case Example

Jessica is a 15-year-old girl with autism and moderate learning difficulties who has a fascination with barcodes and cash tills: she has a collection of seven in her bedroom at home. She is given the opportunity to work in a supermarket for her Year 10 work experience, and does surprisingly well. With the help of her Connexions personal adviser, she is able after she has left school to get an apprenticeship set aside for young people with learning difficulties in a retail store, and is able to stay on in a paid position after the end of the training period.

BOX 32.12 Case Example

Jermaine has a diagnosis of Asperger's disorder and has always been interested in collecting rubbish. When he leaves school, his parents manage to get him onto a college course on environmental studies. He does a module on recycling. This eventually leads him to a paid position in the local rubbish dump ensuring that as many items of rubbish are recycled as possible – a job that he enjoys immensely.

Sensory sensitivity may affect one or more of the five senses – sound, sight, touch, smell or taste. The child's senses may be intensified (*hyper-sensitive*) or attenuated (*hypo-sensitive*).

➤ *Sound* – Many young people on the autistic spectrum find some background noises unbearably loud or distracting. In contrast, most of us automatically filter these out and are usually able to ignore them. Examples include the sounds of: a Hoover, a fan, a washing machine, a washing-up machine or a lawnmower. Discordant, unpredictable or unclear noises may cause a level of distress that appears disproportionate: examples include fire alarms or a supermarket public announcement. Such noises can be experienced as physically painful or can give rise to anxiety – which may at times be overwhelming. Other difficult sounds may include echoes or a room full of people talking.

➤ Certain *lights* may be experienced in the same way. Examples include harsh strip-lights, flickering lights or light bulbs without shades.

➤ Many young people on the autistic spectrum find any form of *touch* acutely unpleasant. One young autistic man has described how every drop of water in the shower feels to him like a painful pinprick. Some dislike the feel of labels on clothes, and cut them off. More generally, touch from another person is aversive.

➤ Others may feel reassured by the touch of certain *textures*; examples include particular fabrics, rubber, bumpy objects, smooth soft things, fringes on cushions, people's hair or ladies' tights. The need for comforting sensations may contribute to stereotypical movements such as rocking, spinning or hand-flapping.

➤ Many of those on the autistic spectrum are nevertheless *hypo-sensitive* to pain or extremes of temperature. Such hypo-sensitivity may be a contributory factor in self-injurious behaviour such as biting or scratching.

➤ *Smells* such as perfumes or adhesives or *tastes* such as garlic may similarly cause severe discomfort.

At *school*, some classrooms may create particular difficulties if they present a combination of sensory difficulties such as echoing sounds, fluorescent lights, the close proximity of others and the smells of the teaching materials used. These difficulties are graphically described from a young person's perspective in the book '*The Curious Incident of the Dog in the Night-Time*'.[11]

Motor incoordination may arise as a result of sensory difficulties or lack of kinaesthetic (body part) awareness. This can make it harder to: navigate rooms, avoid obstructions, keep at an appropriate distance from other people (*see* above, under Social Interaction), and carry out 'fine motor' tasks such as tying shoelaces. Frequently the young person may appear clumsy, as he trips over or bumps into things or people.

Learning difficulties

There is a strong link between generalised learning disability and autistic spectrum disorder. Overall, the more severe the learning difficulty, the more likely there are to be autistic features; and the more severe the autistic condition, the more likely there are to be learning difficulties.[12] The contrary trend can be observed in Asperger's syndrome: young people of high intelligence are more likely to have some features of Asperger's disorder; and young people with Asperger's disorder are likely to be of average or above-average intelligence – but this partly depends on which definition of Asperger's disorder is used and how strictly it is applied.

Exceptional memory

Some young people on the autistic spectrum have an exceptional memory and can recall many facts about a particular subject of interest or the contents of a whole book, film or television programme, especially if it is relevant to a particular skill or obsession.

BOX 32.13 Case Example

A 16-year-old lad with Asperger's disorder takes great delight in greeting staff at his college when they park their cars in the morning. He also likes to look in the visitors' book to see who has signed in. Later in the day when he meets anyone he can tell them the registration number of their car!

PRESENTATION

The expression of autistic symptoms varies throughout childhood, and how the autistic features come to professional attention depends to a considerable extent on the home and school environment. Common stages when autistic tendencies may create problems are at the beginning of any school year, or at times of transition from one school to another (such as primary to secondary, or middle to high). The impact of such life stages may heighten anxiety, lead to an increase in obsessions, or find expression in increased aggression. A behaviourally troublesome child may be seen as merely naughty or rude; an academically failing child may be seen as merely lacking ability; and a verbally competent autistic child who conforms to school rules and is not disruptive may not come to professional attention for many years. This may result in many individuals with Asperger's disorder not being diagnosed until the later years of school, or in adulthood, if ever.

BOX 32.14 Case Example

James seems to be doing very well for most of Year 4, although he has some difficulties in September of that year. At the beginning of October in Year 5, when he is still nine years old, James has a 'complete wobbly' that requires his head teacher to restrain him in his office.

When the educational psychologist looks into the situation, she finds that James had a good relationship with his Year 4 class teacher but clashes with his Year 5 class teacher, and is getting into all sorts of trouble in class. James turns out to have significantly below-average intelligence with some additional specific areas of academic weakness, such as numeracy. He has a number of autistic features. His mother says that he is quite different from his elder brother, who has done well at the same school.

James is given some extra support through the school's own special needs funding and the local Behavioural and Educational Support Team. Year 6 turns out to be a lot easier for James, as he develops a good working relationship with his class teacher.

BOX 32.15 Case Example

Anthony has been placed in a special tutorial unit because of his difficulties attending school. Despite this, he refuses to leave home, and he is just about to start Year 11.

The tutorial unit asks his primary mental health worker to visit Anthony at home, as the last contact the staff had with him suggested that he was unhappy. Anthony does not initially emerge from his bedroom. While they are waiting for him, Anthony's mother explains to the primary mental health worker that Anthony has always been a bit of a loner, but now it seems he is even more reluctant to go out. He rarely eats meals with the family, but prefers to spend time in his room on his computer. He does not always get on with his stepfather or younger half-sister. His mother is worried that he seems very thin and pale.

When Anthony reluctantly emerges, he seems to have poor eye contact, but this is partly because his eyes are covered by his hair. He explains that there is nothing he enjoys at school. After some prompting, Anthony reveals that he likes playing around on his computer, mainly gaming, particularly with role-playing games. He plays mainly on his own, but with one particular game, he plays with a number of others online. Does he communicate electronically with his friends? Anthony says he does a bit.

The primary mental health worker thinks Anthony may have Asperger's disorder and depression, but is not sure. She offers Anthony an appointment with a psychiatrist in specialist CAMHS to discuss antidepressants, but he refuses, and his mother says she is not keen on his having medication. The primary mental health worker discusses Anthony with staff at his tutorial unit, who confirm that he has never been very sociable, but emphasise they have been more worried about his being depressed than having autistic features.

At the follow-up home visit, the primary mental health worker notes that Anthony is spending a bit more time with his family, as he has been allocated a place on the electronic learning programme, which means that the local educational authority has installed a new computer in the family living room, with fast Internet access. He and his mother are quite enthusiastic about this, so no further appointments are arranged.

Anthony's mother subsequently fails to respond to letters offering further home visits, so the case is closed.

BOX 32.16 Summary of the main features of autistic spectrum disorders

Difficulties with social communication and social interaction
- Difficulty identifying emotions in self and others
- Difficulty imagining another's point of view
- Few close or intimate friends
- Usually a preference for being alone and a lack of interest in others; occasionally a thwarted desire to be with others; sometimes both
- Language difficulties, often quite subtle:
  - Construes expressions literally
  - May misunderstand humour, sarcasm, puns or double-meanings
  - May repeat words or phrases without meaning (echolalia)
  - May use certain words out of context, whose meaning therefore jars or is not clear
- Often infrequent or reluctant eye contact; occasionally a tendency to stare
- Problems with turn-taking, reciprocity and two-way communication
- Speech may be unusual in several ways:
  - Monotonous tone
  - Lack of appropriate gesture, facial expression or other non-verbal accompaniment
  - Content dominated by own interests
  - Fulfils a need to express things (rather than a need to share in a two-way conversation)
- Responses to others can appear odd, rude or inappropriate (perhaps as a result of the last four bullet points)

Repetitive behaviours, restricted interests and difficulty with change
- Preference for established routines, which are often idiosyncratic
- Distaste for change, which often leads to anxiety or other forms of distress
- Play is likely to be repetitive and oriented towards objects rather than people
- Although play may be imaginative, it seldom shows social imagination
- The range of interests is likely to be limited and obsessional in character, and not shared with others
- Repetitive, 'stereotypical' movements may occur, such as hand flapping, body-rocking, spinning, finger movements or chewing (these are more common in autism than milder conditions on the spectrum)

TABLE 32.1 Differential diagnosis and prognosis of autistic spectrum disorders

	Classical autism	High-functioning autism	Atypical autism	Asperger's disorder	Autistic spectrum disorder (and none of the others*)	Language delay or disorder
Age at which symptoms begin	Onset before three years	Onset before three years	Usually after three years	There are usually features in the developmental history that make the child different, but suspicions may not arise until primary or secondary school, if ever.	Symptoms become apparent at any stage after three years.	May become apparent as slightly unusual child-parent interaction during the first year, or when language milestones are not achieved.
Age at diagnosis	Usually diagnosed pre-school	Diagnosis is usually before or just after school entry.	Any age	The average age of diagnosis is 11 years or around the time of school transition. Or it may never be diagnosed: adults who may well have the condition often have insufficient difficulties to justify any diagnosis.	Varies	Usually picked-up pre-school. Language disorder should be diagnosed by the early years of primary school, but occasionally is missed.
Distinguishing features	Intelligence quotient varies: 75% are under 70	Intelligence quotient by definition 85 or more	Atypical either because of late onset or due to lack of one	Can have a range of autistic features, but usually with less impairment than in high-functioning autism (but sometimes the	A mixed picture, the most common being a combination of autistic features not meeting a strict diagnosis;	Skills deficit in one or several areas of linguistic competence, including: • expression • comprehension

History of language delay or disorder	There is usually a history of language delay or disorder. There is often a particular skill.	dimension of the core features	two may be indistinguishable apart from the age of onset) May have a particular skill, but often clumsy, or have other associated features	and with too much of either learning disability or language disorder to fit Asperger's.	• social use of language.
Schooling and prognosis	Usually require special educational provision in a school or base for autistic children or for children with learning difficulties. About 10% of affected adults work, often in semi-sheltered settings. Many live at home or in supported accommodation.	Very variable	Special educational needs vary. Mainstream primary or first school should be adequate for most. Middle and secondary/high school may be much more challenging, and some may require more support than can be given in mainstream. After secondary school, life may become easier, especially if a skill niche can be found.	Special educational needs vary. May require special schooling. May present management difficulties, as children or adults, for instance with disruptive or aggressive behaviour.	Children with *delayed language development* usually catch up by the early years of primary school. Management under the guidance of a speech and language therapist may accelerate this. Children with *language disorders* may require support in school, or even placement in a language unit. Some of these will turn out to have an autistic spectrum disorder. A minority will continue to need help in secondary school.

* This is probably equivalent to pervasive developmental disorder not otherwise specified (PDD-NOS).

Different subgroups exist; all encompassed by the term autistic spectrum disorder – or pervasive developmental disorder (which, confusingly, is a slightly broader category, as it includes some rare conditions not usually regarded as being on the autistic spectrum; these rare conditions may be omitted in ICD-11).[13] The main subgroups and their distinguishing features are summarised in Table 32.1.

ASSESSMENT

The following components of assessment, or questions to consider, are likely to contribute to an assessment. Time factors may dictate the need to be selective. Sometimes it is enough to do only the beginning of an assessment in order to decide what to do next.

➤ Who is concerned about what?

➤ What has brought things to broader professional attention *now* (rather than previously or later)?

➤ What problems is the young person having at home, at school or with peers?

➤ If there are several areas of concern (as is likely in autistic spectrum disorder), then make a list. If possible, consider ranking the concerns in order of significance.

➤ Does the child have any other known medical, developmental or mental health problems – such as a genetic syndrome, learning difficulties or anxiety?

➤ Take a *developmental history*. This should include a school history from the first nursery to the present.

➤ What is the current situation at *school*? How is academic progress? How are social relationships? What happens in the classroom? What happens in break times (play sessions and lunch break)? Has there been any teasing or bullying (as victim or perpetrator)?

➤ What assessments have already been done? Has the child ever seen an educational psychologist or a speech and language therapist? Has there been any assessment of academic potential or achievement? What opinions or advice have been given?

➤ Take a *family history*. This should include: the current family set-up, any similar concerns about siblings and any family members with developmental disorders. Is the young person similar to anyone else in the family?

➤ What are parents' ideas about the nature of the problem? (Include if possible the ideas of an absent parent.) If relevant, what are grandparents' ideas?

➤ What do parent(s) hope to achieve from your discussion? Can you help them achieve this?

➤ What strategies have been tried at home and at school?

➤ *Observe* the child. Not all of the observations suggested in Table 32.2 will be possible in a single interview, but it is worth keeping a look out for these sorts of issues.

➤ Does the young person have impairments in each of the *three areas of concern* in autistic spectrum disorders?

TABLE 32.2 Possible elements of observation in suspected autistic spectrum disorder

General	Social communication	Social interaction	Repetitive behaviours, restricted interests and difficulty with change
What does he do while you are talking to his parent?	How does he connect to the content of your conversation? Does he join in appropriately and take turns in conversation? Is the content of his speech relevant to what others are talking about or dominated by his own interests? Does he continue talking about these even when you change the subject or try to talk about something else? Does he respond to your attempts to involve him in conversation only if you talk about the right subject?	How does he respond to his parent(s) during your discussion?	Does he line up toys or sort them according to size, shape or colour?
How does he play with the toys or drawing things available?	What level of language comprehension does he show? Does he appear to understand what is being said? Does he misunderstand expressions or words? Are there some things he takes literally when they are not meant literally?	How does he respond to you (the interviewer) non-verbally during the conversation?	Does he play in an imaginative way, for instance using figures to represent people? If so, do parents regard it as novel or something they observe repeatedly?
	What level of language expression does he show? Does he find it easy to say what you think he might mean? Do you need help from his parent to understand him?	How frequently and comfortably does he make eye contact? Does he stare or look at you in an unusual way?	Does he repeat several versions of the same drawing, or cover a variety of themes?

(Continued)

General	Social communication	Social interaction	Repetitive behaviours, restricted interests and difficulty with change
	Is there anything unusual about the way he talks? For instance, does he speak in a monotone or in a pseudo-adult way?	Does he use gesture and non-verbal communication?	Does he make any unusual movements or gestures? Examples include: flapping when unsure of the answer to a question; picking at a body part; touching, licking or stroking things in a certain way; any repeated movements; or tics (*see* Chapter 25 on Tics and Tourette's syndrome).
	Does he say anything that seems rude or tactless?	Can he see another person's point of view? You can try asking him questions using examples as they come up in the interview: 'What is your mum worried about?' 'What do you think has made mummy upset?' 'How do you think the other boy at school felt when you did what mum just said you did?'	

A brief summary of the salient points of the assessment may be a good way of ensuring you and the family view the situation in roughly the same way: a shared *formulation* (*see* Chapter 3 on Middle Childhood). This can help decide on management.

MANAGEMENT AND REFERRAL

If you suspect an autistic spectrum diagnosis once you have made your own initial assessment, it is usually beneficial for both child and parents if you refer them for a definitive diagnosis to a specialist autism diagnostic service (usually based in specialist CAMHS or community paediatrics). The process of detailed assessment may be very helpful for the family even if the conclusion turns out to be that such a diagnosis is not justified. Rather than refer every child with autistic features, which could clog up a valuable specialist resource, it may be more constructive to do a small amount of further assessment yourself first. In particular, it is worth asking someone in the school who knows the child well whether there are any concerns. If there is nothing from the school's point of view that is consistent with an autistic diagnosis, then it is unlikely that the specialist team will make an autistic diagnosis. Depending on local circumstances, it may be worth referring to speech and language therapy or paediatric occupational therapy before involving the whole specialist team.

Explanation and understanding: sometimes called psychoeducation

Although parents vary in how keen they may be for a diagnostic label, most are grateful for any explanation of their child's behaviour that does not imply it's because of what they are doing wrong. Simple attributions of the child's difficulties may help enormously.

BOX 32.17 Case Example

> When the community school nurse meets with John's mother, Louise, to discuss their joint concerns about John, aged eight years, she knows she will not be able to give anything approaching a diagnosis regarding John's autistic features, as this would need to be multidisciplinary. She finds that Louise is in no hurry for certainty, but is very relieved at the idea that John's dislike of change and preference for routine seems to be a character trait rather than something she is doing wrong. Louise feels guilty about giving into John's demands, but appreciates the explanation that his anxiety is increased by unexpected change. After some discussion, they agree that Louise should try to give John as much warning as possible of any changes to his routine; and that she should try to avoid situations where his anxiety is likely to be increased by changing what he is used to, such as what he wears or what he eats.

The kinds of explanation that may be helpful for parents of children with autistic features (with or without an autistic spectrum diagnosis) include the following.

➤ Share as much as possible of your formulation with a parent or if possible both parents. It doesn't really matter how much uncertainty you are in about what it all means, since you can share this as well – most parents appreciate this sort of honesty. It may be best to do this without the young person being present. Depending on the age of the young person, it may be helpful to direct a simplified version of your summary to him (but make sure you check with the parent(s) first how much they think you should say).

➤ The autistic features are *not* due to any immunisations. There is now abundant evidence of *no* link between the measles, mumps and rubella vaccine and the onset of autistic features, other than their occasional occurrence at roughly the same age.

➤ Some of the child's difficulties may best be understood as a consequence of **language difficulties**, such as misunderstanding or taking things literally. The impact of this may be underestimated if the child has no history of language difficulties and appears to speak fluently. Referral to a speech and language therapist, especially one with a particular interest in the autistic spectrum, may help define the nature of these difficulties. If a speech and language therapy assessment has already been done, it is worth looking carefully at the recommendations to see if these are being followed.

BOX 32.18 Case Example

Mary, a nine-year-old girl with Asperger's syndrome, is often in trouble at school for getting agitated in class and wandering around.

Closer analysis shows that this occurs when her teacher says: 'Wait a minute and I will come and help you'. She waits exactly a minute: if the teacher does not come within that time, Mary gets out of her seat. When asked, she explains how distressed she is that the teacher has *lied* to her.

➤ For some individuals with autism, the **sensory environment** can be quite overwhelming. Hypersensitivity to sounds, smells, touch or personal proximity may make everyday situations into a terrible ordeal: being in a classroom, in a shop, on a pavement or on an underground train can all be unbearable in ways which may be impossible for the individual to explain. Imagine a child who emerges into this sort of sensory onslaught and cannot understand why others do not experience things the same way. An adolescent aged 13 years and several adults have written first-hand accounts of this sort of experience, and how they coped.[14,15,16] An occupational therapist may be very helpful in delineating the extent of the sensory difficulties (which may of course occur in the absence of an autistic diagnosis).

➤ **Positive aspects of having an autistic spectrum disorder** – It is too easy to develop an overemphasis on the negative aspects of autistic conditions. While it is important to acknowledge the challenges of parenting or teaching a child on the autistic spectrum, it is also important for the child, parents and teachers to be aware of the advantages to such a condition. This is not a textbook of evolutionary theory, but it seems to the authors that there must be an evolutionary advantage to such a common condition. Historians may get into debates about whether some famous and successful people had Asperger's, such as Marie Curie, Andy Warhol, Margaret Mead, Glenn Gould, Albert Einstein, Jane Austen and Benjamin Franklin, but there is no substitute for direct contact with the individual, and many of these people had some aspects of genius, which overlaps to some extent with Asperger's. Box 32.19 gives 25 potential advantages for someone with Asperger's disorder. Once the possibility of an autistic diagnosis has been mentioned to a child or young person, it may be helpful to go through this checklist with him, with or without his parents, to find out which characteristics he thinks he has and emphasise the positive aspects of the condition.

➤ There is an increasing profusion of *information* sources about autism and autistic spectrum disorders, some of which are mentioned at the end of this chapter.

Further assessment

Further assessment may be necessary for children whose parents or teachers want to know if a diagnosis is justified. The National Autism Plan for Children[17] makes

TABLE 32.3 Twenty-five potential advantages for individuals with Asperger's disorder

Thinking	With others	General
Meticulous	Guardians of those less able	Organised
Detail-oriented	Open and honest	Independent
Focused	Uninterested in social expectations	Capable of developing strong skills in specific areas
Inquisitive	Witty and entertaining	Enthusiastic about their passionate interests
Logical	Dependable	Finely attuned to their sensory systems
Unambiguous	Loyal	Able to create beautiful images in their mind's eye
Good at word games and play	Rule followers	Able to create beautiful sounds in their mind's ear
Storage banks for facts and figures, with a great long-term memory	Ethical and principled	
Tenacious researchers and thinkers – good at persevering		
Average to above-average intelligence		

recommendations about how assessment should best be carried out, and many areas have built up multidisciplinary (and multi-agency) assessment protocols as a result; in some areas, diagnosis is still led predominantly by a single discipline, usually community paediatrics or child and adolescent psychiatry. The diagnostic process tends to take a long time (often appropriately): the kind of support detailed in this section may be useful during this waiting period.

➤ *Detailed assessment of specific abilities* may be included in the multidisciplinary protocol. If not, it is worth ensuring that the following components are at least discussed as options with parents and/or school.

— *Speech and language therapy* assessment and recommendations

— *Occupational therapy* assessment for either sensory issues and/or motor difficulties

— The child's functioning in school is likely to be affected by his overall intellectual level and the pattern of strengths and weaknesses. These are best assessed by an *educational psychologist* or *clinical psychologist*, depending on local circumstances

— Associated developmental disorders such as neurological or genetic syndromes are best assessed by a *community paediatrician*

— Associated developmental disorders such as ADHD or Tourette's disorder are best assessed by a *child and adolescent psychiatrist* or *community paediatrician*, depending on local circumstances.

Strategies

Autistic features are *not* a consequence of parenting – but some parenting strategies *can* make them easier to cope with – for both the child and his parent(s). Similarly, children on the autistic spectrum respond very well to some strategies in school, but adversely to others.

Simple problem-solving can be used to generate ways of responding more effectively to the sort of difficulties that may arise from autistic features, such as:

➤ increases in anxiety

➤ tantrums of frustration

➤ outbursts of aggression

➤ avoidance of certain social situations

➤ obsessions that interfere with family life.

BOX 32.19 Case Example

Deepak, a 13 year old with Asperger's disorder and co-ordination problems, has always hated sports day, and has become increasingly reluctant to go to school at the end of the summer term. His mother discusses this with the special needs coordinator: together, they decide that this year they will arrange something different for him.

The special needs coordinator suggests that Deepak could be allowed to serve refreshments instead of taking part in races, as she knows he is interested in home economics and catering. When this is discussed with Deepak, he responds enthusiastically. When the day comes, he goes to school early. A catering assistant whom Deepak knows from his classes has been delegated to keep an eye on him, and he enjoys the school sports day for the first time ever.

Visual timetables can be introduced at home or at school, but are particularly useful to help young people cope with the complex sequence of changes characteristic of the school day – more so in secondary than in primary school. These should be individually tailored according to the child's needs, language and ability. The child can be encouraged to join in with making the weekly plan, using his computer expertise if appropriate. Stickers and pictures can be added to personalize this and reflect his individual interests. With a child of low verbal ability, recognisable symbols can be used instead of words.

Sensory strategies: A number of sensory strategies may be suggested. Examples include: brushing the skin, weighted blankets, rocking chairs, chewy tubes, sucking ice and various toys that can be stretched or twirled or fiddled with. Some children like the feeling of a weighted blanket and are more able to settle to sleep or sit still if they have one. Similarly, rocking can be very calming for some. These methods seem able to help some children reach the right state of alertness or relaxation. For sensory overload, simple advice such as the use of headphones to reduce noise or sunglasses to cut out bright light can be very helpful. Referral to an occupational therapist may be invaluable not only to assess sensory difficulties but also to provide detailed ideas for management.

BOX 32.20 Case Example

Sean, a 10-year-old autistic boy with little verbal language, loves his chewy tube. He will spin it, stretch it or chew it, particularly if anxious about being in a novel situation. He always carries it around with him. In familiar environments, he will put it in his pocket. His parents have bought several metres so they can cut a new piece off when he loses the one he has with him.

Dealing with routines and obsessions: Routines can be *functional* – meaning that they help everyone (or most people); or *dysfunctional* – meaning that they have an adverse impact on the child or those around him.

➤ A *morning routine* may serve the function of getting *any* child ready for school. For a child on the autistic spectrum, this can often be very helpful for him, but may perhaps have an adverse impact on everyone else in the household, for instance if the bathroom is blocked for ages. If the routine is taking the child over to such an extent that he is regularly late for school, then it may be dysfunctional for everyone.

➤ A *bedtime routine* may help *any* child settle at night, and even more so a child with autistic traits. If however the routine becomes so prolonged and anxiety-provoking (for instance if any small mistake means that the whole routine has to be restarted from the beginning) then it may be counter-productive.

➤ *Obsessions* at any time of day may become preoccupying and time-consuming.

➤ Obsessional interests can be used as a *reward* for other desired activities.

BOX 32.21 Case Example

> Callum, aged 14 years with a diagnosis of Asperger's disorder, is extremely interested in medieval history: he loves reading books about this.
>
> There are certain school lessons he sees as pointless, such as English: his view is that he can speak it and write it, so why should he have to learn it?
>
> A plan is set up whereby he is allowed to spend 10 minutes at the end of each English lesson reading his favourite medieval history book – but only after he has done the work set. Although he still does not see the point of English lessons, he does begin to do the work set in class.

➤ Obsessional interests can be used as a *calming strategy*, especially if they help to relax or de-stress a child, for instance after his return from school (which many children on the autistic spectrum find much more stressful than most adults think). Time-limited immersion in a favourite activity can be a functional routine, such as:
— bouncing on a trampoline
— drumming
— painting models.

➤ *Limiting the time a child spends on obsessional activities* can be achieved by:
— using timers, so he can see how long he has left to complete an activity
— establishing rules, such as turning off the television or Internet access at 9 pm (parents must stick to the rules they set)
— drawing up a visual schedule (with symbols or pictures) for use at non-school times, which can have on it not only the things that he *has* to do, such as mealtimes, homework and bedtimes, but also the activities he *wants* to do, according to his interests
— including some slots for unplanned or free time, as few families would want to be rigidly timetabled for a whole weekend.

➤ *Tackling unwanted routines and obsessions* may be no easy matter, and may require referral to a clinical psychologist or clinical nurse specialist with skills in cognitive-behavioural therapy. *Distraction* can be very useful at times in diverting a child's attention from the planned sequence. *Firmness* may be necessary in cases of school lateness. But in general, it is not helpful to attempt to counter every example of child rigidity with parental rigidity: this is a recipe for escalating conflict. Parents are unlikely to find it helpful if they hear you saying no more than: 'You should be firmer'. Battles should be selected carefully: it is

really worth fighting only those which matter. In addition to the case of school tardiness, other examples include:
— a child who is so intent on reaching the right shop that he crosses the road without looking
— a child who will not buckle his seatbelt because it presses his clothes against his skin
— a child who would spend his entire waking Saturday on a games console if allowed.

Teaching social skills and mindreading. A number of different approaches can be used to help a young person with an autistic spectrum disorder learn about:
➤ his own thoughts and feelings
➤ the thoughts and feelings of others
➤ how to behave more appropriately in social situations.

Emotional recognition can be taught using drawing exercises with think bubbles or prepared materials such as:[18]
➤ comic strips to make explicit what others are thinking[19]
➤ DVDs such as *Mind Reading* – an electronic encyclopaedia of human emotions and their expression[20]
➤ *The Transporters* – for younger children, using trains with faces on them.[21]

Role play and drama can be useful for some but confusing for others. ***Direct individual or group social skills programmes*** are designed to teach specific rules of social behaviour, such as:
➤ how close to stand to someone else
➤ shaking hands
➤ greeting others
➤ when and how to use eye contact
➤ turn-taking in conversation
➤ how to make small-talk
➤ what to do in awkward situations.

Whilst these can be very effective, some young people have difficulty generalising what they have learnt in the therapy setting to contexts that have not been specifically described.

BOX 32.22 Case Example

Roderick, aged 13 years, is having weekly therapy sessions to help him learn social skills. In session number 23, he reports going up to a stranger in a public urinal and trying to shake his hand. He and his therapist have not until then discussed what to do in public toilets.

If a young person is struggling with a particular social situation, he can be prompted to write a story about it, generating alternative developments and solutions. This technique is called *social stories*.[22,23] The prepared stories include a script aimed at helping the child learn what to expect. These can be used both at home by parents and at school as part of the child's Individual Educational Plan. Combining both approaches is likely to be more than doubly effective, not only providing consistency but also promoting the ability to generalise.

Adaptations of *cognitive behaviour therapy* can be used if the young person has sufficient language and the cognitive capacity to think about his thoughts and responses. The aims may include recognition of the components of anxiety or anger, and developing strategies to deal with them.[24,25]

Parenting programmes or groups are also available specifically for parents of children diagnosed with an autistic spectrum disorder, such as the EarlyBird programme for preschool children and the EarlyBird Plus programme for children diagnosed between four and eight years, both developed by the National Autistic Society.[26]

Specific teaching approaches may be very helpful, despite seeming resource-hungry. A well-established example is *TEACCH (Treatment and Education of Autistic and Related Communication-handicapped Children)*.[27] If this is not available, the child's Individual Education Plan should include strategies recommended by relevant professionals, such as the educational psychologist, speech and language therapist and/or occupational therapist.

Befriending, mentoring, and social support – Although many young people on the autistic spectrum have difficulty making friends, some really want to make new friends or to be included more in social situations. An approach that can help at school is setting up a *Circle of Friends*.[28] Alternatively, a school-based buddy system or the use of peer mentoring may help reduce social isolation and feelings of loneliness – at least at school. Parents can help by encouraging attendance at some form of social activity or after-school club (with extra support if necessary and available). Examples that often work well include chess club, drama club or a martial arts class, but any activity based on the child's particular interests has a good chance of keeping the child involved despite the inevitable social challenges.

Consider all aspects of the school day. For a young person on the autistic spectrum, difficulties are most likely to occur at certain times of day.

➤ *On the way to and from school* – Public transport may present a major challenge for any individual with autistic features to negotiate, but school buses can be an opportunity for bullies to operate unchecked. Walking to school can also present opportunities for victimisation. Cycling to school may present a dilemma for parents who want the child with no traffic sense to be safe and teachers who want the young person to cycle on the road – to protect others. Such a divergence of views can usually be resolved by adequate discussions involving a parent and relevant school staff, perhaps mediated by a professional from a linked agency. (*See* below and Chapter 22 for further comments on bullying.)

BOX 32.23 Case Example

> Gustav is 14 years old and is having some difficulties at secondary school that his mother thinks may be due to Asperger's syndrome, although his teachers are not convinced. They tell him to cycle to school on the roads, as he has passed his cycling proficiency test. His mother, however, is aware that Gustav has not developed an age-appropriate traffic sense, so tells him to cycle on the pavement. Gustav often responds to these contradictory instructions by leaving his cycle at home, walking all the way to school, and arriving late.

➤ *On arrival at school* – Between entry to the school premises and arrival in the classroom there are a number of unpredictable encounters that a young person with autistic features may find challenging. Some children benefit from coming into school early to avoid the hubbub; others may prefer to have a predictable routine, such as reporting to a particular member of staff on arrival, who can then guide the young person through registration and into the classroom.

➤ Other *unstructured times* may also cause difficulties. These may include break times and lunchtimes, and – particularly in secondary school – walking from one classroom to another along the school corridors. Many young people on the autistic spectrum benefit from having the support of a learning support assistant, which may be even more necessary during these unstructured times than it is in the classroom. Others may benefit from spending major portions of the school day in the special needs room, learning support department or library (with staff support).

BOX 32.24 Case Example

> Mina, an eight-year-old girl with Asperger's disorder, has considerable difficulty separating from her mother and coming into school. She creates a great deal of disturbance, kicks and screams, and has to be forced into school. She takes a long time to settle down in the mornings, but later in the day becomes more settled and able to work with her teaching assistant.
>
> Arrangements are made for Mina to come into school via the side of the building, where she is greeted by her teaching assistant, who accompanies her to the classroom in three stages – via a quiet corridor, then the library, then the classroom. If Mina needs to, she is allowed to sit in the library and look at books until she feels calm and able to enter the classroom. Once in the class, she has her own workspace with a visual timetable set in a quiet part of the room. Her teaching assistant is available for her for 15 hours per week: half the school timetable.
>
> With these arrangements, Mina finds it easier to come into school and settle to work, although she still becomes unsettled if she has a supply teacher, if her teaching assistant is off, or after a break from school due to illness or holidays.

➤ Research on **bullying** in UK schools has found that pupils with special needs are more likely to be bullied than other children, particularly in secondary schools.[29] Surveys suggest that nearly two-thirds of children with special needs are bullied compared with just over a quarter of other children: much of the bullying experienced is related to the nature of the special needs. Particular characteristics such as clumsiness or the person's special interests may be used as a pretext for bullying. Often such children do not have protection and support from other children, and the victimisation may occur when school staff are not in the immediate vicinity, so the bullying may continue for a long time unrecognized. Children with an autistic spectrum disorder are particularly likely to overreact and get into trouble themselves, or get into the habit of bullying others. A number of strategies may be useful, including:
  — the provision of some form of support or activity at lunchtime or break times
  — a special room the young person can go to when things are getting difficult
  — a card he can show the class teacher to enable him to go there, and leave the class without having to ask or explain
  — training in assertiveness, social skills, accurate interpretation of others' social overtures and conflict resolution.[30]

Consider whether particular **aspects of learning** might be difficult for the child. This includes not only specific or general learning disability, but also teaching or learning contexts that may be challenging. Examples include the following.
➤ A full psychometric assessment (by an educational or clinical psychologist) should highlight any areas where more help may be needed, as well as areas of strength.
➤ In children on the autistic spectrum, special educational needs often include language difficulties, coordination problems (not necessarily amounting to dyspraxia) and sensory difficulties.
➤ If there is a specific literacy difficulty, then extra time may be needed in exams, or in some cases a scribe.
➤ Older pupils on the autistic spectrum may find the examination situation intolerable: having to sit in a room full of others, the clock ticking, the invigilator walking around looking over her shoulder, the questions being ambiguous. Such pupils may be unable to function if subjected to the same rules as others, so may need special dispensation to sit exams alone, or with only a small number of others, in a familiar and comfortable environment, and possibly with some support to interpret the questions. Others may find the examination situation easier than their usual classes, as rules are applied more strictly, everything is quiet, and nothing unpredictable happens.

Any form of **transition** can be anxiety-provoking for someone on the autistic spectrum. Examples include the following.
➤ **Having a supply teacher for a day** – This will be easier if the supply teacher used for the class is always the same person, and if the pupil has a familiar learning support assistant.

➤ *Moving up a year at school* – This should be easier with adequate preparation, such as meeting the new teacher and visiting the new classroom at the end of the term before the change occurs – possibly several times.

➤ *Moving from one school to another* – This is likely to need more preparation. A pupil on the autistic spectrum may need:

— several trips to his new school in the last term before the change
— detailed consideration of his journey there
— an explanation of his future timetable
— a map of the school
— meeting the special needs coordinator
— meeting any learning support assistants he is likely to have
— getting a cast list of the adults who will be important for him to know in the new school
— meeting a buddy or peer mentor.

➤ *Moving house* – Adequate planning, with repeated visits and discussions, should help with this, but it may be particularly stressful if it is associated with other major changes, such as a move of school or a change in family composition.

Diet

Some parents report improvements in their child's behaviour on wheat-free or dairy-free diets. However, the research trials of gluten and/or casein and/or yeast free diets in autism have so far been inconclusive. Care should always be taken to ensure that the diet is not becoming too restrictive and therefore *nutritionally inadequate* (especially if the child will eat only certain types, colours or textures of food). If there are concerns about the nutritional adequacy of the diet, then refer to a dietician.

Medication

Prescribing may be necessary for co-existing problems such as ADHD, anxiety, obsessive-compulsive disorder or Tourette's disorder. A common problem with children on the autistic spectrum, particularly those with below-average intelligence, is **aggressive behaviour**: this can become more manageable with a low dose of risperidone, such as 0.5 mg once or twice per day. Weight gain is often a significant problem, in which case other similar medications may be tried, such as aripiprazole. The use of orodispersible (melt-on-the-tongue) or liquid preparations may be helpful for children who have difficulty swallowing tablets.

Some children with developmental disorders have intractable *sleep* problems and may benefit from the use of melatonin at night. The dose required may be greater for younger than older children: a starting dose is usually 2 mg, but this can be gradually increased – if there is no response – up to 20 mg. Side effects are uncommon with this approach, but may include headache, dizziness, nausea, restlessness, itching or an increased heart rate.

RESOURCES
Websites
- The National Autistic Society has much information and advice, including books and resources for families, individuals and education staff: www.nas.org.uk
- A charity called Research Autism lists every known intervention and gives each a rating: www.researchautism.net
- The American website www.autism.fm – based at Yale University – gives up-to-date information on research and other informative websites.

Books for children
- Bleach F. *Everybody is Different*. USA: Autism Asperger Publishing Co; 2002.
  This book is for siblings of a child with an autistic spectrum disorder.
- Chilman-Blair K, Taddeo J, Baron-Cohen S. *Medikidz Explain Autism (Superheroes on a Medical Mission)*. London: Medikidz Foundation; 2010.
  One in a series of UK books in graphic novel format explaining childhood disorders to children.
- King-Smith D, Bailey P. *The Crowstarver*. London: Corgi Childrens; 1999.
  This is a moving story of a foundling raised by a shepherd in Wiltshire in the 1920s who turns out to have autism and learning difficulties but an 'idiot savant' capacity for mimicking and communicating with animals.

Books for parents
- Atwood T. *The Complete Guide to Asperger's Syndrome*. London: Jessica Kingsley; 2008.
- Atwood T, Andron L. *Our Journey through High Functioning Autism and Asperger Syndrome: a roadmap*. London: Jessica Kingsley; 2001.
  This book describes the ways autistic disorders affect families' daily lives, and how to overcome these challenges, using stories from families who have agreed to share them.
- Baron-Cohen S. *Autism and Asperger Syndrome (The Facts)*. Oxford: Oxford University Press; 2008.
- Howlin P. *Autism and Asperger Syndrome – Preparing for Adulthood*. London: Routledge; 2004.
- Vermeulen P. *I am Special: introducing children and young people to their Autistic Spectrum Disorder*. London: Jessica Kingsley; 2000.
  This is a workbook designed for children with Autistic Spectrum Disorder to work through with a parent, teacher or other professional – in groups or individually. It explains how to inform a young person he is on the autistic spectrum in a positive way by covering his potential strengths as well as the difficulties he may face.
- Wolkmar FR, Wiesner LA. *A Practical Guide to Autism: what every parent, family member, and teacher needs to know*. New York and Chichester: John Wiley; 2009.

REFERENCES
1 McGilchrist I. *The Master and his Emissary: the divided brain and the making of the Western world*. London: Yale University Press; 2009.
2 Lord C, Rutter M. Autism and pervasive development disorders. In: Rutter M, Taylor E, Hersov L, editors. *Child and Adolescent Psychiatry: modern approaches*. 3rd ed. Oxford: Blackwell; 1994.

3 www.psych.org/MainMenu/Research/DSMIV/DSMV/DSMRevisionActivities/DSM-V-Work-Group-Reports/Neurodevelopmental-Disorders-Work-Group-Report.aspx

4 Bertrand J, Mars A, Boyle C, *et al*. Prevalence of autism in a United States population: the Brick Township, New Jersey, investigation. *Paediatrics*. 2001; **108**(5): 1155–61.

5 Baron-Cohen S, Scott F, Allison C, *et al*. Prevalence of autism-spectrum conditions: UK school-based population study. *British Journal of Psychiatry*. 2009; **194**: 500–9.

6 www.cdc.gov/mmwr/preview/mmwrhtml/ss5810a1.htm

7 World Health Organization. *The ICD-10 Classification of Mental and Behavioural Disorders: diagnostic criteria for research*. Geneva: World Health Organization; 1993.

8 Williams E, Thomas K, Sidebotham H, *et al*. Prevalence and characteristics of Autistic Spectrum Disorders in the ALSPAC cohort. *Developmental Medicine and Child Neurology*. 2008; **50**(9): 672–7.

9 Bondy A, Frost L. The picture exchange communication system. *Behavior Modification*. 2001; **25**(5): 725–44.

10 Russell AJ, Mataix-Cols D, Anson M, *et al*. Obsessions and compulsions in Asperger syndrome and high-functioning autism. *British Journal of Psychiatry*. 2005; **186**: 525–8.

11 Haddon M. *The Curious Incident of the Dog in the Night-time*. London: Vintage, 2004.

12 Fombonne E. The changing epidemiology of autism. *JARID*. 2005; **18**(4): 281–94.

13 www.who.int/classifications/icd/ICDRevision/en/index.html

14 Jackson L. *Freaks, Geeks and Asperger syndrome: a user guide to adolescence*. London: Jessica Kingsley; 2002.

15 Grandin T, Scariano M. *Emergence: labeled autistic*. New York, NY: Time Warner International; 1996.

16 Williams D. *Somebody Somewhere: breaking free from the world of autism*. London: Jessica Kingsley; 1998.

17 Le Couteur A. *National Autism Plan for Children*. London: National Autistic Society; 2003.

18 Howlin P, Baron-Cohen S, Hadwin J. *Teaching Children with Autism to Mind-read*. New York, NY: Wiley; 1999.

19 Gray C. *Comic Strip Conversations: illustrated interactions that teach conversation skills to students with autism and related disorders*. Arlington, TX: Future Horizons Inc; 1994.

20 www.jkp.com/mindreading

21 www.thetransporters.com (developed with the Autism Research Centre at Cambridge University)

22 Gray C, McAndrew S. *My Social Stories Book*. London: Jessica Kingsley; 2003.

23 Gray C, Arnold S, Pauken S. *The New Social Story Book*. Arlington, TX: Future Horizons Inc; 2000.

24 Attwood T. *Exploring Feelings: anxiety: cognitive behaviour therapy to manage anxiety*. Arlington, TX: Future Horizons Inc; 2001.

25 Attwood T. *Exploring Feelings: anger: cognitive behaviour therapy to manage anger*. Arlington, TX: Future Horizons Inc; 2001.

26 www.nas.org.uk/earlybird

27 www.nas.org.uk/teacch

28 www.nas.org.uk/circleoffriends

29 Sharp S, Smith PK. *School Bullying: insights and perspectives*. London: Routledge; 1994.

30 Sharp S, Smith PK. *Tackling Bullying in your School: a practical handbook for teachers*. London: Routledge; 1994.

CHAPTER 33

Developmental disorders, Part 3: Speech and language[1]

INTRODUCTION

Terminology

Communication is a multifaceted process, which can be regarded as beginning before birth. It consists of the transmission and receipt of information via verbal or non-verbal means. The foetus communicates to the mother by growth and movement; the mother in return by containment and nourishment. Later, an element of understanding is generally considered important. Concerns about a child's smiling or establishing eye contact may arise within the first few weeks of life. A responsive baby melts everyone's heart. It is a matter of debate how much understanding the baby is doing, but, when it is there, the reciprocation is unmistakable.[2]

Perhaps the most common concern to reach professional attention is about delay in learning to talk. Parents may seek advice from other family members, friends, the child's health visitor, playgroup leader, nursery teacher or class teacher about this. The constituent skills involved in learning to talk are staggeringly complex, and it is amazing that most humans, in contrast to animals, manage to achieve this ability.

Speech is the oral production of sounds to aid communication. **Language** is the encoding of meanings in words (spoken and written) and non-verbal signals. **Non verbal communication** includes facial expressions, gesture, eye contact and posture.

There are traditionally four components to language.[3]

Phonology refers to the ability to produce and discriminate the specific *sounds* of a given language (*phonee* means voice or sound; *logos* means word, science or study of).

Grammar refers to the underlying rules that organise any specific language. It can be divided into **morphology**, the within-word structure, and **syntax**, the between-word structure (*syn* means together and *tassein* means to arrange).

Semantics refers to meanings (*sema* means sign and *semantikos* means significant). A partial measure of semantic skill is the size of a child's **vocabulary**, which is relatively easy to assess informally. Vocabulary includes both concrete and conceptual items. By 24 months of age, the average child knows 50 words. A young child can acquire up to 10 new words per day. Early use of gesture and subsequent size of vocabulary both correlate with school and social success.[4] Early childhood environments impoverished in adult-to-child communication can significantly disadvantage the child, so parents should be encouraged whenever possible to gesture, speak and read to each of their children at every opportunity – from birth onwards. Semantic difficulties may involve misunderstanding the meanings of some words, particularly those that are ambiguous or sound the same. An example might be 'berth' on a ship misunderstood to be 'birth': 'We are going to have a berth on the ferry to Spain' … 'Oh, I didn't know you were expecting another baby!' Some children with semantic difficulties may find words describing abstract ideas more of a challenge than words describing concrete objects; this tends to be more difficult to spot. An example could be the child who can understand what 'blushing' means but has more difficulty with the concepts of 'shame' or 'embarrassment'.

Pragmatics refers to the development of skill in communicating (*pragma* means deed and *pragmatikos* means practical). Conversation has implicit rules, such as turn-taking, topic maintenance and conversational repair. There are also unspoken rules about politeness, storytelling, talking for a long time, and signalling what you intend to say. This also includes the child's ability to understand how the meaning of any word may vary with context and in relation to the speaker's intention. *Prosody* refers to the use of stress (on a word or a syllable) and tone of voice – and the interpretation of the meaning this adds to what is said (*prosoidia* means a song sung to music or the tone of a syllable).

Speech and language may be *delayed* or *disordered*. Delays are much more common than disorders. In **delay**, the sequence of development is unaltered, but *everything is later than expected*. In **disorder**, there is an *abnormal sequence* of development.

Speech disorders affect the way speech is produced, for instance by the lips, tongue, cheeks or larynx. Some examples follow.

➤ **Dysarthria** means literally a difficulty (*dys*) articulating or making the movements necessary for speech, or more simply just unclear speech (*praxis* means action). It can be due for instance to cerebral palsy.

➤ **Hypernasality** – a very nasal tone of voice – can be due to cleft palate.

➤ **Stammering** is a disturbance of the fluency of speech, with hesitations, prolongations and repetitions of sounds within words: it is called **stuttering** in North America and Australia. Children whose maturity of thought outstrips their maturity of speech production may repeat themselves or trip over words as they try to get thoughts out. Some children may become anxious about this, which can then lead to an established problem; there may also be genetic factors.

➤ **Speech sound disorders** affect phonology (so overlapping with language) and may make it difficult for children to be understood. They can take various forms, which are usually consistent in all that the child says:
  — **omissions** – leaving out sounds or syllables
  — **additions** – adding an extra sound or syllable to a word
  — **distortions** – getting a sound wrong
  — **substitutions** – saying one sound instead of another.

Language disorders affect the central processing of verbal ideas and communication, and can present with effects mainly on phonology, grammar, semantics or pragmatics – or some combination. Two broad subgroups include *expressive* (difficulty *producing* language) and *receptive* (difficulty *understanding* language).

BOX 33.1 Case Example

Timothy is three-and-a-half years old when he is taken into care due to neglect by his mother Abigail, who has schizophrenia. He is noted to have extreme expressive language delay, uttering no more than single words.

There is debate in the court hearing for the Care Order about whether or not this is due to neglect. Abigail argues strongly that she has a strong family history of boys being late to speak. Investigation by a community paediatrician into other family members, with the full cooperation of Abigail and other relatives, reveals that there are three other boys on mother's side of the family with expressive language delay, just as Abigail said.

However, none of them had such bad delay as Timothy's, and he has many other features of neglect, so the judge grants the Care Order.

Timothy is subsequently looked after by his paternal aunt, since his father seems unable to safeguard him. In the aunt's household, Timothy's speech and language make rapid progress.

Specific language impairment is called 'specific' because it is not just a consequence of other developmental disorders, such as global (overall) developmental delay, neurological impairment or autistic spectrum disorder; *and* to signify that it is impaired to a greater extent than other aspects of intelligence. It includes both delay and disorder. It can also be called: *developmental language disorder*, meaning that it affects specifically the development of language; *dysphasia*, meaning that it is a difficulty (*dys*) with speaking (*phanai* means to speak); or even *aphasia*, meaning that certain aspects of language are just not there (*a* means not).

Normal development

A simplified account of the stages of language development is shown in Table 33.1 – to be read with the understanding that, as with most of child development, there is a great range of normal variation.

Some factors influencing language development are shown in Box 33.2.

Abnormal development

The term *'speech delay'* applies in practice both to difficulties at the level of speech production and to delayed phonology development. Delays in the maturation of speech sounds usually normalise by the age of nine years: residual errors persisting after this age affect approximately 5% of the population. There may be a family history.

TABLE 33.1 Population-based norms in language development

Stage	Age
Babbling	6–10 months
Word comprehension	8–10 months
Word production	12–13 months
Word combinations: telegraphic speech first: ('daddy-car' instead of 'daddy's car')	14–24 months
Grammatical development	24–30 months
Basic morphology and syntax	By age 3 years

In six to seven year olds, *specific language impairment* occurs in 6% of girls and 8% of boys.[5] Latest figures from the Bercow Review show that 7% of five year olds entering school have significant speech, language or communication difficulties; 1% have severe difficulties.[6] Children can also present with speech, language or communication difficulties secondary to other difficulties such as autism, cerebral palsy, hearing loss and learning difficulties.

TABLE 33.2 Factors influencing language development

Within the child	Environmental
Genetic – There is often a family history of similar problems, a common example being expressive language delay (*see* Case Example in Box 33.1).	**Family size** – On average, children from larger families are slower to speak. This is most likely to be due to the reduced interaction with adults each is likely to have.
Gender – Girls are generally more advanced in early language development than boys.	**Parent–child interaction and communication** – The more the better for the development of language.
Twins speak on average a bit later than singletons. This is probably because they have to share parental attention, so they get less each; or possibly because they can satisfactorily communicate non-verbally with each other, so they have less need to develop verbal communication.	**Neglect** can be strongly associated with delayed language development – which may improve greatly in a more stimulating environment (*see* Case Example in Box 33.1).
Medical conditions may delay language acquisition. One common example is *deafness*, the commonest cause of which is glue ear (which can lead to language delay – especially receptive – if recurrent or persistent). Language may also be delayed due to *global developmental delay*, whether the cause is known or unknown.	**Bilingual upbringing** – Although it used to be thought disadvantageous to confuse children with two sets of vocabulary and grammar, it is now clear that children taught two languages from before the age of two years are at no disadvantage, and may experience considerable advantages as adults.

Deficits in the development of *pragmatic* skills are common in autistic spectrum disorder, when they are often combined with *semantic* difficulties. Examples include disregarding context and taking things literally, such as: 'Pull your socks up' or 'Every cloud has a silver lining'. Because of their common co-occurrence, the term *'semantic-pragmatic disorder'* was coined to describe a group of children with this combination of problems – who were originally thought *not* to be autistic. There is continuing (and perhaps fruitless) debate about whether or not such children should now be seen as fitting on the autistic spectrum.

Selective mutism (also called *elective mutism*)

These terms refer to a child who is silent in some situations but not all. When she does speak, language development appears normal. It is considered to be more of an emotional than a developmental disorder, in that *situational anxiety* appears to be the driving force in at least a proportion of cases.

When she is silent, the child may communicate with gestures or by nodding, pushing or shoving. It is usually at playgroup, nursery or school that the mutism presents, with some initial shyness, and perhaps some *selective* conversation with one or two people. Conversation at home is usually adequate, although even there the child may speak with only a select group of people.

Selective mutism is more likely to develop in children who are temperamentally shy and prone to anxiety. There may be a history of language delay in the first 2–3 years of life; some affected children may have an underlying learning disability. It is slightly more common in girls than boys and occasionally develops following a traumatic event.

Treatment consists of trying to create an environment at home and school that encourages and reinforces *all* attempts at communication and independence and avoids reinforcing the mutism.[7]

BOX 33.2 Case Example

Sophie, aged five years, has been in her Reception class for six months. Her class teacher has become increasingly concerned over time about Sophie's communication. When she started in proper school, Sophie appeared very shy and anxious. Given that she was then not yet five, the teacher thought this was understandable, and would improve with time as Sophie settled in. It has not: as time has gone by, it has become increasingly apparent that Sophie does not speak in the school environment (the classroom, the playground and the dining room). She is however adept at using non-verbal communication skills such as nodding, pointing and smiling.

Sophie's parents are surprised by this behaviour, as Sophie is able to talk freely at home and also in other environments such as friends' houses and shops. They have observed Sophie at children's parties, where she has been reluctant to engage in any activities.

With full support from Sophie's parents, the class teacher asks the school's speech and language therapist for her advice about how to encourage Sophie's verbal communication in school. Following her assessment, the speech and language therapist discusses with Sophie's parents a graded program to help her make progress in small steps. The first step is for her parents to invite a chosen class friend around to play at home: in that context, Sophie is able to speak freely. Then other friends are invited home.

After Sophie demonstrates being comfortable speaking at home with several of her peers, her parents shift the context to the local park: again Sophie is able to speak clearly. The next step involves Sophie's mother being present at similar play dates with just one or two peers in the school playground, and then inside the school building. Once Sophie appears confident about talking with a couple of peers inside a room in the school with her mother present, the next step is to substitute a learning support assistant for her mother – who is able to withdraw gradually. The learning support assistant is then able to introduce fun games that simulate occasions when verbal communication is required in the classroom. These games are then replicated within the classroom.

By the time Sophie reaches the end of Reception, she is able to respond verbally at registration and speak to her class teacher when in small groups, although she is still silent during activities involving the whole class. Improvement continues as Sophie moves up the school.

Relevance to child mental health
Delay or disorder in speech or language is strongly associated with:
➤ behavioural problems[8]
➤ other developmental disorders, such as:
  — speech sound disorders
  — reading disability.[9]
➤ child mental health disorders.[10]

Looking at this the other way round, 62% of children with identified child mental health problems in one study had speech and language difficulties, just under half of which had been previously identified.[11] This implies that at least 50% of children presenting with mental health problems may have unidentified speech and language problems. Young offenders have also been found to have high levels of speech and language difficulties as well as unrecognised specific or general learning difficulties, ADHD, conduct disorder and substance misuse.[12]

What is the nature of the link between language disorders and mental health problems? As with many other aetiological questions, there are four possibilities, described as follows.
➤ *A causes B* – Common sense suggests that children who cannot say what they are thinking are likely to get frustrated; and that children who cannot understand what adults say to them are also likely to get frustrated – and not obey the adult. It is difficult to see how a child with inadequate language could express frustration

directly: he is hardly likely to say 'I am frustrated'. Children are liable therefore to express frustration in a variety of non-verbal ways, including for instance:

— as an emotional (***internalising***) disorder, such as anxiety, withdrawal or unhappiness
— as a behavioural (***externalising***) disorder, such as oppositional defiant disorder, conduct disorder or delinquency.

➤ ***B causes A*** – Internalising difficulties such as sadness, anxiety or post-traumatic stress disorder and externalising difficulties such as ADHD may include as part of the way they manifest:

— ***regression*** to an earlier stage of development – a four year old, for instance, may start talking in baby language
— not being able to put words together coherently – ***expressive*** difficulties
— not listening to what adults say or taking then in – ***receptive*** difficulties
— not being able to understand the point of view of the speaker – ***pragmatic*** or theory of mind difficulties.

➤ ***C causes both A and B*** – Some brain disorders and genetic disorders may cause *both* a language disorder *and* a child mental health problem – the mediating factor sometimes being generalised learning disability.

➤ ***Different perspectives*** – Whether the problem is seen as A or B depends on who is looking at it. The timber merchant, the botanist and the artist do not see the same tree. A disorder of social communication may be seen:

— by a speech and language therapist as a language disorder
— by a psychologist as a developmental disorder (affecting more than just language)
— by a teacher as a behavioural problem
— by a parent as 'Just like uncle John' or even 'Just like I was as a child'
— by a child psychiatrist as a psychiatric problem.

There may be validity to each of these perspectives, but there may be a danger for the child in assuming all are equally valid (a position sometimes described as *social constructionism – see* Chapter 8 on Family Issues). For instance, to attribute a six-year-old boy's antisocial behaviour to his parents' lax attitude and anti-authoritarian stance, while it may have some truth, can significantly disadvantage the child if it obscures professional recognition of underlying difficulties such as a specific literacy difficulty, a speech and language disorder, a developmental motor disorder, an autistic spectrum disorder or ADHD. At best, this could be described as doing an incomplete assessment; at worst, it could be regarded as professional negligence.

ASSESSMENT AND REFERRAL

For this reason, when you are asked to see a child whose speech or language is the main concern, cast your net as wide as possible, and ensure your curiosity extends to any possible causative or co-existing disorder (*see* Table 33.2).

The single most important of these to think of is ***deafness***: any assessment of language delay or disorder *must* include a hearing test – if one has not already been done. A distraction hearing test may sometimes miss hearing loss, in which case pure-tone audiometry may be required. When in doubt refer to the local audiology service: staff at this clinic will *not* consider you are wasting their time![13]

BOX 33.3 Case Example

Jermaine is referred at seven years of age by his general practitioner to the primary mental health worker because of concerns about his behaviour. When asked who is most concerned, his mother explains that she can manage him at home, but he is very disruptive in the classroom. The primary mental health worker notices that Jermaine's speech seems a little indistinct, and asks whether his mother has any concerns about this.

To her amazement, Jermaine's mother says, 'Well, not really: I was told when his deafness was diagnosed that he would be a bit behind with his language' There is nothing about deafness in the referral letter.

The primary mental health worker arranges a school meeting involving the class teacher, head teacher and mother. It emerges before this is held that the head teacher has received a copy of the letter from the audiology clinic detailing the full nature of Jermaine's hearing difficulties, but has filed this, and the class teacher is unaware of Jermaine's deafness. The primary mental health worker gets the impression from her telephone conversations with teaching staff that they are not fully aware of the impact of deafness and language delay on behaviour, and have related Jermaine's behaviour to his mother's tendency to be aggressive when she should be assertive. Jermaine's mother is quite open about this, and explains it as a consequence of her white working-class upbringing. There may also be an element of covert racism (Jermaine's father, whom he no longer sees, is black Afro-Caribbean).

At the school meeting, everyone is able to discuss Jermaine's difficulties in a calm and constructive fashion. His deafness is not bad enough to justify input from the peripatetic teacher for the deaf, but the head teacher agrees to put him on the special needs register, and allocate to him some learning support assistant sessions.

It is important to be aware of any additional medical problems, such as delays in other areas of development. Potential associated mental health problems have been mentioned above, and may need attention in their own right, perhaps even more importantly if *not* attributable to the speech or language difficulty. There may be important aspects of the family to consider.

➤ Is there enough stimulation – from parents, siblings, grandparents and other family members?
➤ Could there be neglect, emotional abuse or domestic violence?
➤ What is the family's first language?
➤ Are there ethnic or cultural issues?
➤ How has the family engaged with professional networks, such as the health visitor, playgroup, nursery school and school?
➤ Which professionals if any are currently involved?

A child with language delay due to an established cause, such as the boy described in Box 33.3, may not need to see a speech and language therapist (or may already have seen one), but many children presenting with speech or language difficulties may need this sort of specialised assessment, particularly if it is not clear whether the child has a disordered sequence of development or merely delay. Whether or not you should make this referral depends partly on past and present professional input. For instance, if the child is already being seen by a local community paediatrician for concerns about possible developmental delay, then such a referral would be superfluous. Occasionally, a speech and language therapist may already be involved without the parents being fully aware (although they should have been told), for instance indirectly via school or through a special needs nursery, in which case you will not achieve added value by referring again.

MANAGEMENT

Although a child with *delay in language development* is likely to catch up, this process can be accelerated by appropriate help – from those adults he spends most time with.

➤ Delayed *comprehension* can be managed by carers simplifying how they speak to the child, and introducing new concepts by linking them with what they are about – rather than testing the child with questions. In such cases, adult stimulation can help the child develop age-appropriate language, so that speech and language therapy may not be needed.

➤ Delayed *expression* can be managed by carers modelling the correct way for the child to say things – rather than correcting errors constantly. For instance, a child with normal hearing and otherwise normal development who says 'gog' for 'dog' will pick up the correct pronunciation after hearing it often enough.

➤ If the structure of sentences (*syntax*) is delayed, speaking to the child in slightly longer sentences will allow the structures to be absorbed and reproduced.

A child with *disordered language development*, in contrast, should be seen by a speech and language therapist. The therapist's assessment will usually end with a discussion of the implications for the child's learning and academic progress at school; he will usually make recommendations about ways in which school staff and parents can help the child. Some children may require direct speech and language therapy.

Parents of a child with a *stammer* should avoid laughing at him, making him self-conscious, or increasing his anxiety in other ways. This will give the child time for his language skills to catch up with his thinking. If the problem is clearly more than transient, or simple advice along these lines is ineffective, early referral to a speech and language therapist is advisable – to avoid the anxiety becoming so established that it leads to a persistent problem. A chronic stammer may also be an index of other anxieties, or the expression of emotional difficulties, which may need help in their own right.

REFERENCES

1 We are indebted to T. Boutwood, Specialist Speech and Language Therapist, Bournemouth and Poole Teaching Primary Care Trust, for her contribution to this chapter.

2 Gopnik A. *The Philosophical Baby: what children's minds tell us about truth, love and the meaning of life.* London: The Bodley Head; 2009.

3 Toppelberg CO, Shapiro T. Language disorders: a ten-year research update review. *Journal of the American Academy of Child and Adolescent Psychiatry.* 2000; **39**(2): 143–52.

4 Rowe ML, Goldin-Meadow S. Differences in early gesture explain socio-economic status disparities in child vocabulary size at school entry. *Science.* 2009; **323**(5916): 951–3.

5 Tomblin JB, Records NL, Buckwalter P, *et al.* Prevalence of specific language impairment in kindergarten children. *J Speech Lang Hear Res.* 1997 Dec; **40**: 1245–60.

6 Department for Children, Schools and Families. *The Bercow Review: a review of services for children and young people (0-19) with speech, language and communication needs.* London: Department for Children, Schools and Families; 2008. Available at: www.johnbercow.co.uk/bercowreview (accessed 2 April 2011).

7 Keen DV, Fonseca S, Wintgens A. Selective mutism: a consensus based care pathway of good practice. *Arch Dis Child.* 2008; **93**(10): 838–44.

8 Tomblin JB, Zhang X, Buckwalter P, *et al.* The association of reading disability, behaviour disorders and language impairment in second-grade children. *J Child Psychol Psychiatry.* 2000; **41**(4): 473–82.

9 Pennington BF, Bishop DV. Relations among speech, language and reading disorders. *Annu Rev Psychol.* 2009; **60**: 283–306.

10 Goodyer IM. Language difficulties and psychopathology. In: Bishop DVM, Leonard LB, editors. *Speech and Language Impairments inCchildren: causes, characteristics, intervention and outcome.* Hove: Psychology Press; 2000. pp. 227–44.

11 Ibid.

12 Bryan K, Freer J, Furlong C. Language and communication difficulties in young offenders. *Int J Lang Comm Dis.* 2004; **42**(5): 505–20.

13 Hall D, Williams J, Elliman D. *The Child Surveillance Handbook.* 3rd ed. Oxford: Radcliffe; 2009.

CHAPTER 34

Developmental disorders, Part 4: Motor development[1]

INTRODUCTION

Look at most textbooks of child mental health and you will be lucky to find more than a few lines on motor problems such as **dyspraxia** (*dys* means difficult and *praxia* means action or coordinated movement). You are likely to have the same problem with textbooks of neurology or child development. It is as if motor inco-ordination is treated as *someone else's problem* – rather like children's mental health, in fact. The 'someone else' in this case is the paediatric occupational therapist. So why are we trying to write something about this when it's obviously their job?

The answer is that there is a strong association between all sorts of problems in motor development and child mental health problems. It would be nice to follow this statement with a table of which motor problems correspond to which child mental health difficulties. Unfortunately, it would be impossible to construct such a table: each child seems to have *a different combination of difficulties*. The most that can reasonably be said as a generalisation is that if a paediatrician or child mental health professional expects most children with a motor difficulty to have a single, easily definable problem, then she is likely to be disappointed.

This observation used to be encapsulated in the idea of '**minimal brain damage**', which was hypothesised to give rise to a number of different subtle difficulties with movement, coordination, attention, language, learning and social development. This was a lovely idea, because it seemed to explain so much. There was one crippling problem with it: there was no confirmation of the hypothesis. In most such children, no clear evidence of brain damage was found, other than the presenting symptoms. So it was pure presumption to conclude that these symptoms were a consequence of some unidentified 'damage' – due to factors unknown. It was also a pejorative presumption, and one that became politically incorrect.

The 'minimal brain damage' concept was then replaced by a supposedly value-free label: **DAMP**. This stands for a 'Deficit in Attention, Motor control and Perception' – or alternatively a 'Disorder of Attention, Movement and Perception'.[2]

➤ The **A** refers to ADHD, with or without hyperactivity. Debatably, the symptoms may fall short of a categorical diagnosis.

➤ The **M** refers to the sort of problems that are the subject of this chapter, namely developmental motor coordination disorder, otherwise known as developmental coordination disorder, **dyspraxia** or clumsiness. Presenting symptoms include frequently dropping things, poor performance in sports and poor handwriting. There may simply be delay in motor development rather than disorder, but if so this is out of proportion to any delay in other areas of development. An affected child tends to have not only impairment or immaturity of certain movements but also impaired *organisation* of movement – and also difficulty organising other tasks. The combination of being both clumsy and disorganised can be very frustrating for child, parents and teachers. Whether due to delay or disorder, the motor deficit tends to improve with age. Disordered movement due to neurological diagnoses is excluded from this, for instance:

— cerebral palsy
— traumatic brain injury (*see* Chapter 38)
— muscular disorders such as muscular dystrophy, dystonia or spinal muscular atrophy.

➤ The **P** refers to a heterogeneous group of difficulties, usually agreed to fall short of severe learning disability (an intelligence quotient below 50), but often overlapping with specific or general learning disability (*see* Chapter 35). This group of deficits principally includes:

— specific reading disability – sometimes called dyslexia (*dys* means difficulty and *lexia* means reading) – and often combined with specific spelling disability
— specific language impairment (*see* Chapter 33)
— autistic features, sometimes but not necessarily amounting to a categorical diagnosis of autistic spectrum disorder (*see* Chapter 32).

One way of making sense of this conceptual minefield is to consider each of these different dimensions as a continuum, as in Figures 34.1 to 34.4.[3]

Any one child may be at any point on each of these lines – which can explain why so many children do not fit neatly into simple descriptions or single diagnoses. On the other hand, there probably *are* children with dyspraxia who do *not* have significant degrees of ADHD, specific learning disability *or* autistic spectrum disorder.

All these problems may lead to – or at least be associated with – the following groups of problems.

➤ *Academic impairment* (*see* Chapter 35)
➤ *Emotional impairment* such as:

— poor self-esteem
— being a victim of bullying (*see* Chapter 22)
— school refusal (*see* Chapter 21)
— depression (*see* Chapter 26).

➤ *Antisocial behaviour* and delinquency (*see* Chapter 30).

This may further complicate the way in which the child presents to child mental health professionals. The behavioural or emotional features may **mask** the underlying physiological deficit.

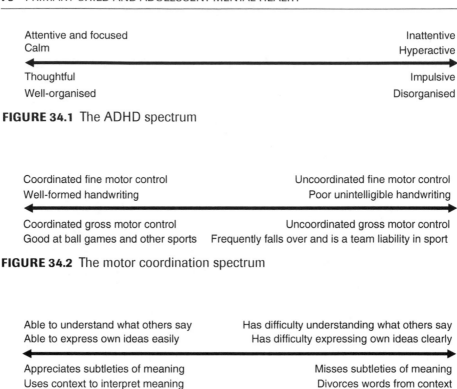

FIGURE 34.1 The ADHD spectrum

FIGURE 34.2 The motor coordination spectrum

FIGURE 34.3 The language spectrum

FIGURE 34.4 The autistic spectrum

ASSESSMENT AND REFERRAL

In view of the likelihood of a range of problems, an overall assessment is important.

The assessment of the *motor component* of the child's difficulties depends on the age. For a child under five, referral to the local Child Development Centre is probably the best option: he is then likely to be seen at least by a *community paediatrician* and a *paediatric occupational therapist*. Once over the cut-off age for referrals to this team, these two referrals may need to be made together, or else starting with whoever seems more appropriate initially.

For a school-age child, *preliminary assessment* could include asking him to:
➤ write something
➤ copy a circle
➤ cut out the paper delineated by the circle
➤ copy a different shape or picture
➤ hop on one leg
➤ walk on the lateral aspects (outside bits) of his feet
➤ put coins in a box
➤ put pegs in a board
➤ catch a soft ball that you throw at him.[4]

It may be as well not to pretend you are an expert in this area (unless you *are*, for instance through being a paediatrician or occupational therapist).

Referral to *specialist CAMHS* is probably justified if you think that the situation is particularly complicated, but not if this could lead to the child's physiological difficulties being overlooked.

MANAGEMENT

Management depends on the nature and severity of the child's difficulties, so it is important to ensure that the full extent and nature of the child's impairments have been adequately explored before launching into explanations of what is wrong or suggestions as to how to help the child.

Psychoeducation can be very important. Many parents, children and professionals find the label of dyspraxia or the hotchpotch idea of DAMP useful, despite finding the initial associations of this word discomfiting. Everything that has a name is less frightening than the unmentionable. To say that a child should not himself be told until older is probably unwise, as it is likely that peers, siblings, parents or other relatives have already pointed out to him at least his clumsiness, if not also his poor concentration and learning problems – in a way that may have made him wonder what is wrong with him. It can benefit some families to have a label that encompasses all the child's symptoms, particularly if these are many and varied – even if this doesn't explain very much. It is important to emphasise that it is neither the child's fault that he finds things difficult nor anyone else's. An additional advantage of thinking of dyspraxia, the DAMP label, or the continuum idea, presented visually in Figures 34.1 to 34.4, is that this can result in children receiving adequate attention to difficulties with movement, language or literacy that can otherwise easily be overlooked – particularly when professional attention is focused on the child's ADHD or behaviour.

Paediatric occupational therapists may be able to provide *direct* remedial treatment on a group or individual basis, in school or in a health setting; or *indirectly* via school staff. As well as improving skills, they are concerned with *maintaining* any skills the child may have. Group interventions (in either school or clinic) may take a sensori-motor approach, which means improving sensory processing in order to develop motor skills. Remediation may focus on:

- ➤ muscle strength
- ➤ body posture (often crouched and awkward)
- ➤ body image (usually distorted)
- ➤ sensory issues
- ➤ fine motor dysfunction, including for instance:
  - — pencil grip
  - — tying shoe laces
  - — eating properly.

Improving skills in these areas may provide the child with a much-needed boost to his self-esteem.

Support in school may help the child reach his potential, in addition to implementation of any recommendations from the occupational therapist. Attentional difficulties may be improved by altering seating arrangements, providing regular reminders of what to do next or ensuring the child has regular prompts to stay on task. Sometimes it may be sufficient for the class teacher to be informed of the full nature of the child's difficulties; other children may need individualised support, most cost-efficiently provided by a learning support assistant.

BOX 34.1 Case Example

Jeremy is six years old when his parents decide to do something about the clumsiness they have been concerned about since he was three. They have been hoping he would grow out of it. One of the reasons for seeking help at this time is that Jeremy seems to be finding it much more difficult than his peers to make his writing at all legible, and is always the last to be picked for team sports. They are not sure who would be best able to provide help, so, having discussed things with Jeremy's class teacher, they visit their general practitioner.

She discusses with them the possible avenues of referral, including community paediatrics, paediatric occupational therapy and specialist CAMHS. Jeremy's parents are surprised at the mention of mental health, but the general practitioner explains that it is very common to have a low opinion about yourself when you are clumsy, and that there is a strong link with language difficulties and ADHD. Jeremy's parents say that he does sometimes seem to misunderstand things, but they thought it was just his age; and, come to think of it, he is rather hyperactive: they thought it was 'just Jeremy'.

After discussing all this, Jeremy's parents opt for a referral to a community paediatrician, in the hope that he or she will be the best person to decide who else should see Jeremy.

When Jeremy and his parents meet with the community paediatrician, he takes a full history and does a very thorough examination. Jeremy has in fact been booked into a joint clinic (for possible dyspraxia) with the occupational therapist, who is therefore able to see him the same day. After comparing their findings, the paediatrician and occupational therapist feed back their conclusion that Jeremy's fine and gross motor difficulties both fall within the lowest 5%, but outside the lowest 1%. So he could be said to have mild dyspraxia.

Jeremy and his mother are booked into a group treatment programme that is due to start in five weeks' time, and which still has some vacancies. The paediatrician agrees to write to the school for a report, asking in particular about symptoms of ADHD, academic progress and language skills.

At the follow-up appointment in three months' time, Jeremy tells the paediatrician that he enjoyed his brain gym. The paediatrician asks him how he got on with other children. Jeremy says they were OK. His mother adds that Jeremy seemed very relieved to meet others who had similar problems, and she found it very helpful to meet mothers of other children with a range of problems, some very like Jeremy's.

They discuss the school report. Jeremy's class teacher has commented that he is struggling to keep up with the work the rest of the class is doing, although he is good at answering questions during class discussions. It seems to be partly his writing that is holding him back, but also he really needs to make much more effort to concentrate and stay on task! She is not aware that he has any difficulty with understanding things or expressing himself. With the benefit of this report, and going through the diagnostic criteria for ADHD with Jeremy's mother, the paediatrician makes a diagnosis of ADHD. He explains that they could either start medication straight away, which he would recommend – as Jeremy is evidently under-achieving in class – or they could get a speech and language assessment first, which he thinks is most likely to be normal – but he can't be sure until it is done. Jeremy's mother says his father is not keen on the idea of medication, and she would rather they get the language looked at first.

Both parents attend the next appointment in six months' time. The speech and language therapist has noted Jeremy's difficulty concentrating. Once he got used to her, he was very chatty but had difficulty sticking to the tasks she set him. His receptive and expressive language and grammar are within normal limits, and her brief assessment of the social use of language suggested that this too is normal for Jeremy's age. Jeremy's parents therefore reluctantly agree to a trial of stimulant medication. The occupational therapist joins them briefly and says she has discussed Jeremy with his class teacher and has arranged for him to have some specific help with his fine motor skills from the learning support assistant already in his classroom. Coming after the group treatment, this leads to improvements in not only handwriting but also other areas. For instance, Jeremy gets better at dressing himself and using cutlery without making a mess.

Subsequent follow-up appointments reveal that Jeremy is making much more progress with academic work, seems to feel better about himself, and has invited several friends home; but physical education is still his least favourite lesson.

RESOURCES

- Stein SM, Chowdhury U, editors. *Disorganised Children: a guide for parents and professionals.* London: Jessica Kingsley; 2006.
- The Dyspraxia Foundation: www.dyspraxiafoundation.org.uk

REFERENCES

1 We are indebted to Amelia Kerswell, Occupational Therapist, Dorset Healthcare University Foundation Trust, for her contribution to this chapter.
2 Gillberg C. Deficits in attention, motor control and perception: a brief review. *Arch Dis Child.* 2003; **88**: 904–10.
3 This idea has been developed (with her approval) from a presentation given by Sue Horobin, Paediatric Occupational Therapist, Wolverhampton Primary Care Trust.
4 Gillberg, op. cit.

CHAPTER 35

Specific and generalised learning disability

INTRODUCTION AND DEFINITIONS

A number of different terms are used to describe people with a learning disability, including for instance learning disabilities and impairments, intellectual disabilities, mental handicap, mental retardation, global developmental delay or developmental disabilities. *Learning disability* refers to a *generalised impairment in intellectual functioning of a long-standing nature*. It is usually associated with impaired functioning in the domains of social and self-care skills. It used to be referred to in the UK as 'mental handicap'. In the United States the term 'mental retardation' is still used. All three terms are roughly synonymous with *levels of intellectual functioning at least two standard deviations below the population mean*.

The educational term *learning difficulty* is roughly synonymous with the above but has a different set of sub-classifications. The rationale for the current terminology is:

➤ it focuses on important interventions, particularly educational
➤ it avoids the term *mental* with its connotation of mental illness (which most people with learning disability do not have), and therefore carries less stigma
➤ it avoids the assumption of immutable handicap
➤ this is how individuals like to be referred to
➤ it can describe specific learning difficulties rather than assuming a global delay.

Different services such as social care, health and education have different Intelligence Quotient (IQ) cut-off points or functional criteria used to determine whether an individual can access the service. This can cause confusion for families and professionals.

Generalised and specific learning difficulty

Generalised learning disability is usually diagnosed when the IQ is less than 70. This applies to approximately 2–3% of the population. *Specific learning disability* (also known as specific learning difficulty or specific developmental delay) is usually diagnosed when there is a particular skill deficit in relation to the child's overall IQ. Examples include expressive language disorder (*see* Chapter 33 on Speech and Language); specific difficulties with writing (*dysgraphia*); specific difficulties with mathematics (***dyscalculia***) and specific literacy difficulties, usually with a combination of delays in reading, spelling and writing (***dyslexia***). ***Dyspraxia*** (developmental motor coordination disorder) may also affect learning skills, for instance by impairing handwriting or self-esteem.

BOX 35.1 Case Example

At the age of eight years, Harish struggles to keep up with his schoolwork and is becoming very disruptive in the classroom. His class teacher is concerned about his reading; his parents insist on a referral to the school's educational psychologist, as they suspect he may have generalised learning difficulties – because the umbilical cord was wound tightly around his neck when he was born. Attainment testing confirms that he is three years behind his chronological age in reading and spelling. His overall intelligence is, however, found to be within the normal range (estimated intelligence quotient between 86 and 98). Harish is reluctant to write anything at all in class, or even at home, and his handwriting seems immature. He is referred to an occupational therapist, who finds that he has developmental difficulties with his fine motor skills.

Harish's parents conclude that that he has both dyslexia and dyspraxia. They put pressure on the school and the local education authority, which eventually results in Harish having a full assessment of educational needs before his transfer to secondary school. His educational statement provides him with small-group literacy teaching, some one-to-one teaching in the Learning Support Unit, and some help in mainstream classes from a Learning Support Assistant. The statement allocates funding to buy him a laptop on which he can do his class work and homework. He is allotted a scribe for his exams who also reads out his exam questions for him.

Medical and educational terminology

In medical terminology, ***mild*** learning disability is in the IQ range 50–70, ***moderate*** 35–50, ***severe*** 20–35 and ***profound*** below 20. There is confusion here between medical and educational terms. The medical term ***mild learning disability*** corresponds to the educational term ***moderate learning difficulties*** (IQ 50–70: roughly 2% of the population). The educational term ***severe learning difficulties*** covers the remaining categories, below an IQ of 50 (roughly 3.5 per 1,000). Hence some special schools are designated for pupils with moderate learning difficulties, some for those with severe learning difficulties and some for both.

BOX 35.2 Case Example

Jerome is referred to the speech and language therapist at the age of three years as he seems to have difficulty pronouncing some of his words. She finds that he has a combination of a speech difficulty (problems with certain consonants) and a language difficulty (problems with expressing himself and with understanding others). Despite continuing speech and language therapy input to his nursery school and primary school, Jerome's problems do not make the expected improvement.

As a child, his mother attended a special school for moderate learning difficulties (IQ 50–70) and his elder sister currently attends the same school. He is also sent there initially, but his behaviour continues to deteriorate. He is subsequently placed in a special school for behavioural, emotional and social difficulties, where it emerges that both his apparently low intelligence and his difficult behaviour may be a consequence of his severe continuing speech and language difficulties. He responds to small group teaching, a highly structured behavioural programme, and increased input from the speech and language therapist: his behaviour improves significantly, and he starts to make slow but gratifying academic progress.

The rest of this chapter will focus mainly on children with generalised learning difficulties, which we will generally abbreviate as 'LD'. Whilst children with specific learning difficulties (which can be abbreviated as SpLD) are also at increased risk of developing behaviour or emotional problems and of having a neuro-developmental disorder, addressing their specific difficulties is the role of the educational system and advice should be sought from educational psychologists, specialist teachers and other educational staff. Input from speech and language therapy is required for speech or language difficulties, and from occupational therapy for possible sensory or motor difficulties such as dyspraxia.

BOX 35.3 Case Example

At the age of nine years, Natasha's general practitioner refers her to the primary mental health worker because her parents are concerned about her defiant and oppositional behaviour, and her increasing victimisation of her six-year-old brother.

Natasha's parents explain to the primary mental health worker that she seems particularly difficult to manage when she returns home from school and on Sunday evenings. The primary mental health worker is puzzled by this, and asks Natasha what she likes about school. Natasha says that she most enjoys playtimes and physical education lessons. She reveals that she does not have many friends in her school year but enjoys very much playing with her younger cousins at weekends – both of which her parents confirm.

The primary mental health worker thinks that Natasha probably has oppositional defiant disorder, and considers suggesting that her parents attend the local behaviour management group for parents, but as part of her assessment she speaks by telephone to Natasha's class teacher. It emerges that Natasha is very quiet in the classroom, and not at all a behavioural problem in school. The primary mental health worker then enquires about Natasha's attainments, which she asks the class teacher to fax to her. These reveal that Natasha is about two years' behind in all her attainment tests.

With permission from the school's educational psychologist, the primary mental health worker arranges for Natasha to have a psychometric assessment by a psychology assistant, supervised by an experienced clinical psychologist working in specialist CAMHS. Natasha cooperates well with the test, concentrates well, and seems to enjoy the individual attention, but becomes frustrated at times. The four subtests of the WISC-IV (Wechsler Intelligence Scale for Children, version IV) give roughly similar scores, showing that Natasha's overall IQ is in the range 64–72.

The psychology assistant feeds back the results of this test to Natasha's parents, who also discuss the implications with the primary mental health worker; with their permission, the primary mental health worker informs the school special educational needs coordinator, who then puts Natasha on the special needs register at the level of 'School Action Plus'. Natasha consequently receives extra help within the classroom from shared teaching assistants and is given a differentiated curriculum, meaning that she has easier work than her peers.

Natasha becomes a lot happier in her last two years of primary school – as does her brother, who no longer gets so badly bullied by her. Six months after the original referral, Natasha's parents tell the primary mental health worker that, now that they understand the nature of Natasha's problems, they are far more sympathetic to her difficulties. She still finds it very difficult to tolerate her younger brother catching her up socially and academically, so their parents have arranged separate after-school and weekend activities for both of them, which keep them happily apart for much of the week.

In secondary school, Natasha spends half her school week in the learning support centre and gets significant extra help in her mainstream classes. She manages without a statement of educational needs.

AETIOLOGY

The distribution of IQ within the population is shown in Figure 35.1. The distribution does not follow a normal curve – there is an additional bump at the low IQ end which represents those children with moderate to profound learning disability. Mild (IQ 50–70) and moderate-to-profound (IQ < 50) learning disability have differing causes and implications.

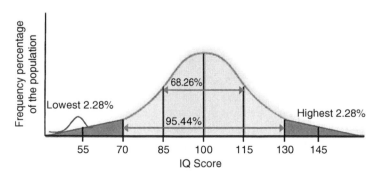

FIGURE 35.1 The normal distribution of scores for intelligence quotient

Intellectual functioning in people with *mild learning disability* is on a continuum with those of normal IQ – since it is the thick part of the tail of the normal distribution. They often have one or more of:

➤ a family history of below average intelligence (sometimes with 'assortative mating', which means that adults of a similar IQ are likely to get together, and some couples may have children, whose IQ is likely to be influenced by the IQ of their parents)

➤ socio-economic deprivation

➤ parental neglect and/or abuse.

The tapering end of the tail of the normal distribution comprises individuals with *moderate-to-profound learning disability*. In contrast to the above group, their parents are usually of average intellectual ability. The children usually have a specific cause for their marked intellectual impairment, which may be:

➤ a chromosomal abnormality such as Down's syndrome which may manifest with characteristic dysmorphic features (40%)

➤ a specific genetic abnormality which affects brain development adversely such as Fragile X syndrome (15%)

➤ an abnormality arising during the pregnancy or perinatal period such as congenital infection, foetal alcohol syndrome, or birth trauma (10%)

➤ postnatal causes such as meningitis, encephalitis or head injury (10%)

➤ undetermined (25%): this is the group many parents find it most difficult to come to terms with; it is sometimes referred to as 'global developmental delay of unknown origin'.

ASSOCIATED PROBLEMS

As well as the LD, the child (and his family) may have a number of associated problems that are either directly related to the condition causing the LD or arise secondary to the LD.

Medical

As LD can often be due to a damaged or malformed brain, it may often be associated with impairing medical conditions, such as epilepsy (*see* Box 35.4) or cerebral palsy (*see* Box 35.5). These may in their own right contribute to the increased risk of developing behavioural or emotional difficulties, and may add to the difficulties faced by the family. Common childhood problems may be harder to detect and manage, especially if the child has impaired communication. Chronic constipation, ear infections, toothache or other childhood ailments may present with a change in behaviour and be missed because the history is unclear or the symptoms are attributed to other causes: for instance, an increase in tantrums may be attributed to the underlying LD when it is in fact due to glue ear and the resulting deterioration in communication; or worsening behaviour may be attributed to increasing academic pressures at school when it is at least partly due to a build-up of constipated stool in the rectum.

BOX 35.4 Case Example

As Frank's epileptic fits become more frequent and harder to control, his development seems to fall further behind, and his behaviour becomes more difficult to manage. He is diagnosed at the age of three years with a complex form of epilepsy involving several different types of seizure. His consultant paediatrician tries him on several different anticonvulsants before finding a combination that seems to provide some degree of control, but EEGs (electroencephalograms) confirm her clinical impression that he is still having frequent seizures, and she needs to adjust the medication frequently as Frank grows older.

Frank goes to a nursery school for children with severe learning difficulty, where staff finds his behaviour difficult to manage at times. He receives his educational statement by four and-a-half years, and goes to a primary school for children with severe learning difficulty. His parents find his behaviour challenging to manage, especially when his epilepsy is less well-controlled. They benefit from support from a social worker in the social care children's disability team and a community nurse specialising in LD, who helps Frank's parents with occasional bouts of targeted behavioural treatment. As Frank grows older and stronger, his family appreciates the provision of respite care in a residential unit managed by social care.

At the annual review of Frank's statement when he is 14 years old, the gathered professionals discuss future plans with Frank's parents. He will have to transfer to a different school when he is 16: his parents want a school in a neighbouring borough, but the local education authority states that one of their own schools would be quite appropriate. Frank's parents seek help from the parent partnership service; with the support of their consultant paediatrician, community LD nurse and disability social worker, they eventually obtain the school of their choice.

Frank's parents remain concerned about his future, as they are not sure they can continue to manage him at home as they themselves get older. Frank's father is due to retire just before Frank's 19th birthday so resolves to devote his retirement to caring for Frank at home. Frank also has two older sisters, one of whom helps her parents with the constant supervision necessary to look after Frank.

Frank never becomes capable of paid employment. When he is 25 years old, Frank moves into a community home with round-the-clock resident carers.

BOX 35.5 Case Example

Ameera's health visitor refers her to a community paediatrician because she has not started walking by 18 months. The community paediatrician diagnoses her as having cerebral palsy of spastic diplegia type, meaning that her legs are stiff (hypertonic) and unable to bear her weight. With the help of physiotherapy and later surgery, she learns to walk short distances, but still requires support for long walks and tends to use a wheelchair more often than not.

A Griffiths test at four years is in the normal range, and she is placed in a mainstream school with support for her mobility; she does not require a statement. On first meeting Ameera, many people assume she must have learning difficulties, but in fact her intellectual ability and academic attainments are within the normal range. Ameera has some difficulties as a teenager making and keeping friends, as she cannot get around independently.

She obtains four GCSE passes and goes on to sixth-form college to study childcare and development. Unfortunately, she is allowed to do only the first year: she cannot progress to a nursery nursing course, as she is not thought safe to carry a baby. She asks to switch to bakery, but an occupational therapy assessment done at the college shows that she cannot remove the baking trays from the oven unaided, as she is not strong enough on her feet, and the ovens are too high for her when she is in her wheelchair. She therefore switches to leisure and tourism, and becomes in due course a hotel receptionist.

Neuro-developmental

There is a huge overlap between LD and the different neuro-developmental disorders (*see* Chapters 31 and 32, Developmental Disorders Parts 1 and 2): children with LD have increased rates of autistic spectrum disorders and ADHD (*see* Figure 35.2) and of Tourette's (*see* Chapter 25 on Tics and Tourette's syndrome).

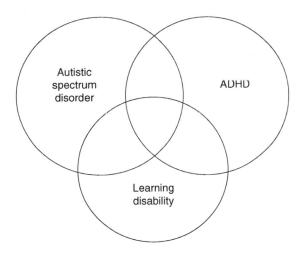

FIGURE 35.2 The overlap between different neurodevelopmental conditions

Effects on the family

The effects on the family should never be underestimated, even in those families who appear to be managing well. Parents may experience a range of emotions, at the time of diagnosis and subsequently, including the following:

➤ initial *relief* at receiving an explanation for the child's difficulties
➤ a sense of *loss* for the 'normal' child they do not have
➤ *denial* (a universal coping mechanism that should not be denigrated)
➤ *anxiety* about the implications, in the present and future
➤ *anger* that it is they who have been singled out
➤ '*chronic sorrow*' about the child's repeated failure to meet age-related norms
➤ *acceptance* of the extent of the disability.

Denial or anxiety may make it difficult for parents to hear or understand the explanations given at the time of first diagnosis. Parents require frequent repetition and elaboration of suitable information as their understanding develops. Different members of the family (mother, father, grandparents, siblings) may work through these feelings at different rates or get stuck at different points. They may require help to work through these feelings, all of which are a normal part of the grieving process.

Ideally, this process should lead towards an **adaptation** to the child and his LD. Many families have an amazing capacity to do this and develop an intuitive understanding of their child and his individual needs. Parents can adjust their career expectations and home lives around their child so that his needs are prioritised.

This may however have an adverse effect on the parents' **own needs** and the needs of **siblings**. Some parents may find the new roles required are very fulfilling; others may become exhausted or depressed. Some may find their couple relationship strengthened; others may find it fractured. The family's combined activities and leisure may be limited by the priority given to the child with LD, who may require much more time and attention than his healthy siblings, whose emotional and social needs can consequently be overlooked.

Economic hardship may result from a parent giving up a job. Practical assistance in exploring the benefit system may help in significantly augmenting the family's income, for instance through the Disability Living Allowance or Carer's Allowance.

Once parents have become fully aware of their child's difficulties, they may be able to **accept** the lifelong commitment. Intellectually, this may help them cope. Emotionally, it may be quite a burden. Events that rekindle awareness of their child's differences from others, and the loss of the anticipated and hoped-for ideal child, may cause a recurrence of some of the grieving feelings described in the first five bullet points above (a process described as '**chronic sorrow**'). A parent may experience fluctuations in mood, which may be linked to the degree of acceptance of the child's disability. At these times, further help may be valuable: sympathetic support and basic practical advice may often be sufficient (see below).

A particularly difficult time for families often occurs when the disabled child reaches the age when other people's children are thinking about **leaving home**, for college, university or full-time employment. Fortunately, special education is a statutory responsibility of local education authorities until the individual is 19 years old. Even so, there is often a gap in provision after the age of 16 years. Parents may become acutely concerned about the young person's capacity for independence, and who will ensure he is cared for when they are too old. There is frequently psychological conflict within the individual's and parents' minds between the need for continuing dependence and support on the one hand, and the drive towards independence and autonomy on the other. Siblings may feel under pressure to provide future care, whether this pressure comes from the parents or from their own beliefs and attitudes.

Social effects

The social complications of having a child with learning disabilities may include:
- less time to leave the home
- less disposable income to spend on leisure activities
- feeling afraid to go out in public due to the affected child's behaviour or language
- feeling misunderstood by others or experiencing stigma
- having less in common with erstwhile friends
- a diminished social life for siblings
- loss of friendships and increasing social isolation due to a combination of the above factors.

BOX 35.6 Case Example

Cynthia is 12 years old when her parents ask their general practitioner for help with her behaviour. She is the middle of three sisters and developed meningitis as a six month old, leaving her with moderate-to-profound learning disability. She has recently started at a secondary school designated for severe learning difficulty. Her parents are finding it increasingly difficult to manage Cynthia's violent outbursts, particularly as these are often directed at her younger sister or their mother.

The general practitioner asks the primary mental health worker to meet with Cynthia and her parents to decide what, if any, additional services might be required. The primary mental health worker witnesses how difficult communication can be with Cynthia, who has only a small vocabulary, and relies partly on sign language to communicate with her parents. Cynthia's periods have recently started, and she is already as tall as her mother. The primary mental health worker obtains descriptions of her challenging behaviours at home, and obtains consent to contact Cynthia's school.

Cynthia already has a social worker in the children's disability team who has arranged for her to have respite in a residential unit for one night per week and one weekend per month, with occasional extra days and nights during school holidays. The social worker is concerned about the physical safety of Cynthia's eight-year-old sister, whom she has met with their 14-year-old sister at their home. Both sisters express a great deal of affection for Cynthia but describe how impossible they find it to keep her calm at home, and how difficult Cynthia makes life for the whole family.

In the absence of a children's LD CAMHS service, there has been no behavioural management offered, but the community paediatrician has tried risperidone. This unfortunately caused excessive weight gain and galactorrhoea (a milky discharge from Cynthia's nipples), so it was stopped. Cynthia's parents refuse to try any other medication. Staff at Cynthia's school, where the community paediatrician does a clinic, tell the primary mental health worker that her behaviour is challenging, but is of a sort the staff are used to dealing with. The school LD nurse has spoken several times to Cynthia's parents and suggests they follow some of the same behavioural strategies that work in school, but the parents seem to find it difficult to work together.

The primary mental health worker, who fortunately feels comfortable with learning difficulties, discusses with Cynthia's parents in her absence how they might be able to deal with this challenging situation. She presents to them the alternatives of being firmer and more consistent with Cynthia or requesting for her a residential school placement. Cynthia's parents seem very anxious about the prospect of sending her away. The primary mental health worker realises this is unlikely to be an issue she can resolve within a few sessions. She discusses referring the family to specialist CAMHS, perhaps for family therapy, but Cynthia's parents are reluctant, as they have formed the impression that the primary mental health worker understands Cynthia and are underwhelmed by the lack of a children's service within CAMHS dedicated to LD.

After discussion with her manager, the primary mental health worker therefore continues seeing Cynthia's parents and occasionally Cynthia herself. It emerges that her parents have grown apart as a result of trying to manage all three daughters, and this makes any sort of cooperative parenting very difficult. They do not want to separate, but want to work things out between them. Cynthia continues to show acts of unpremeditated aggression, directed particularly at her mother and younger sister. The primary mental health worker discusses with her manager, Cynthia's social worker and her head teacher the possibility of a boarding school placement. To the primary mental health worker's surprise, the main resistance to this idea comes not from the multi-agency funding panel, but from Cynthia's parents. They consider they should not abandon Cynthia to the state, and that it is their duty to continue looking after her themselves. They feel extremely guilty about the prospect of 'giving up' on her.

Over the course of the next two years, the primary mental health worker continues to discuss with Cynthia's parents their overwhelming guilt. Eventually, they decide they will themselves bring up the issue of a residential school at the statement annual review. This is then discussed by representatives of health, education and social care at the multi-agency funding panel. A suitable school is proposed. Cynthia and her parents go to visit it. To her parents' surprise, Cynthia enjoys the visit, and they can see that she will be very well looked after there, and will have more appropriate activities and stimulation than at the social care respite centre. They agree to her going there the following September. They explain to the primary mental health worker what a tremendous relief this decision has been to them. They also confide in the primary mental health worker that they have grown closer together again, and are now functioning much more effectively as a couple. They still find Cynthia's behaviour very challenging to cope with, but have found ways of keeping their youngest daughter safe, and think they will probably be able to manage Cynthia during the school holidays, providing the respite care remains available.

At the final follow-up session, after a break of six months since the previous appointment, Cynthia's parents tell the primary mental health worker that they are now getting on much better and feel as if they have rescued their marriage. Cynthia is happy at her new school and her sisters are much happier at home. The holidays are rather stressful, but both parents say they are now coping much better with the difficulties Cynthia presents, and agree that they have at last made the right decision on how best to meet Cynthia's needs.

Educational effects

Due to a political and cultural trend towards social inclusion, only a minority of children with LD now attend a special school (compared for instance to several decades ago). Many children with an IQ below 70 may attend a mainstream school, which for some may be an educational and social challenge that can in itself lead to unhappiness and difficult behaviour. They should have an *Individual Education Plan* or IEP, which is a planning, teaching and reviewing tool setting out:

➤ what should be taught
➤ how it should be taught
➤ whether the pupil requires any additional or differential teaching, such as support from a teaching assistant or withdrawal into small group teaching for literacy
➤ the attainment targets to be achieved
➤ how well the targets are achieved.

It is the responsibility of the Special Educational Needs Coordinator or SENCO to oversee this process.

Some children with more severe or complex needs will have a *Statement of Special Educational Needs* (often referred to simply as a 'Statement') which summarises the child's needs and the educational provision required to meet them. The Statement should also specify any medical or psychological needs and how these are to be met, if necessary from other agencies such as speech and language therapy, occupational therapy or specialist CAMHS. The Statement is reviewed annually. Different local education authorities vary in the amount of help they will give to children without a Statement, but special educational needs support is in general available, up to a certain level, without a Statement.

Parents often find they have to fight hard to get their children's special educational needs met. It is a sad truth that, in a randomly rationed welfare state, parents who are able to persist in fighting for their child's needs in an assertive and articulate way will get those needs met in the end, whereas other parents may not. Parental rights are built into the laws pertaining to educational and social welfare provision. Children who have a Statement of Special Educational Needs are most likely to receive the sort of education they are entitled to, but even they may need parental pressure at the time of the annual review to ensure that provision remains appropriate. In many areas, this process is helped by the provision of free advocacy and support services, often called 'Parent Partnership', which can avert adversarial battles between parents and local authorities.

Effects on mental health (and behaviour)

Children with LD are at increased risk of developing a mental health or behavioural problem. These can be difficult to spot and may be dismissed as being part of the LD. The prevalence rate of mental health problems in young people with LD is over a third compared to 10% in non-LD.[1] Such children are likely to have multiple and complex problems.

Children with any form of LD are at increased risk of developing behaviour that is challenging for their parents and teachers. The behavioural problems range from eating, sleeping or toileting difficulties to severe self-injury or aggression that presents a risk to others. Behaviour is particularly likely to be challenging in some subgroups of LD, such as severe LD, impaired communication or autistic spectrum disorder. A common pattern is of impulsive violent outbursts of verbal or physical aggression that can lead to the sort of anxiety in carers that makes children feel even more out of control.

Children with LD are at increased risk of *child abuse*. This may be for a number of reasons:
➤ the child may be a disappointment to carers, who may not have worked through the anxiety or anger arising from the disability
➤ the child may be exasperating for carers
➤ the child is less likely to take evasive action
➤ the child is less likely to be able to explain convincingly what has happened, or to be believed.

Assessment

Bearing in mind all the above associations, it can sometimes be hard to know *where to begin*.
➤ Who is concerned about what?
  — Is it the parents, teachers or young person himself who is concerned?
  — What are they concerned about?
  — What has prompted these concerns now?
  — What do they want from you or other agencies?
➤ If there is more than one problem, list them.
➤ Is each presenting problem new or old?
  — An acute change in behaviour suggests a medical problem such as pain, infection or other illness; or the development of anxiety or depression. Some autistic children may react with an acute behavioural change to a seemingly minor alteration in routine, such as the class teacher being unwell for a day and replaced by a supply teacher.
  — A chronic problem may be related to a change in psychosocial circumstances. Examples include a parent spending more time away from home through work; or a sibling having a baby.

> What is known about the child?
>   — What is his usual level of functioning?
>   — How does he communicate?
>   — How is he getting on at school?
>   — Does he have one or more diagnoses?
>   — What other medical problems does he have?
> Ask about the family.
>   — Who is at home?
>   — Who does most of the looking-after?
>   — Does the main carer have support from other family members, at home or from within the extended family?
>   — Do the carers have support from friends, support groups or professionals?
>   — Are the parents stressed or exhausted or depressed?
>   — What impact does the index child's disability have on his siblings? Are any of them involved in caring for him?
> What interventions or supportive strategies have been tried?

Then think about which of the presenting problems it might be best to target first, how this might be addressed, and who within the broader family or professional network may be best able to provide the help that is needed.

MANAGEMENT

Parents of children with moderate-to-profound learning difficulty may deal principally with specialist services, but may turn to primary care when they are dissatisfied with the help they are getting, or at an earlier stage when they require referral. Parents of children with mild learning difficulty or specific learning difficulties may suffer from a lack of recognition of their child's needs or a shortfall in provision, or both. It is therefore helpful to have a notion of the sorts of difficulties such children and their parents may experience.

Practical support

This can be provided in a variety of ways.

> Social services may be able to provide *respite care*, either with specialised foster carers or in a residential unit for children with (moderate-to-profound) learning difficulty. Short breaks such as a weekend or one night per week (including the journey from and to school) can allow parents and siblings to have some time without the disabled child. Such alternative care settings are also important for the child with LD, to educate him about different living arrangements and differing routines, thereby encouraging greater flexibility of lifestyle.
> *Direct payments* may be made, which the parents can then use to purchase care for their child.
> *Allowances* and *benefits* are available, such as the Disability Living Allowance and Mobility Allowance. Parents may need help to explore what is available and fill in the often labyrinthine forms, for instance from the Citizens' Advice Bureau or charities such as Contact-a-Family.

> Parent *support groups* can be invaluable, but are not suitable for everyone.
> Other *voluntary organisations* have a patchy distribution, but are often able to fill the gaps left by statutory organisations in meeting the needs of children with LD.

It is therefore helpful to know what is available locally, as well as being aware of national organisations that provide support and advice such as Contact-a-Family and the National Autistic Society (*see* 'Resources' below). Many of these have local branches that parents can join if they wish.

Behavioural management advice

The same techniques can be used as for children without LD. These can be *more* effective with lower IQ, as children are less likely to work out a way around any parental stratagem, and will also not get bored so soon, for instance with a sticker programme. For children with moderate-to-profound learning difficulties or language impairment, the techniques need to be adapted accordingly, and parents may need encouragement to persist with any behavioural programme for long enough to see an improvement. It is often inappropriate for parents of children with LD to join a group of parents who have children without LD, and behavioural sessions may need to be carefully individualised, frequent and continued for a long time.

Advocacy

The lower a child's IQ, the less likely he is to be able to represent his own views and stand up for his own rights. In general, the child's carers will function as his advocate, but there are situations in which this may not happen. If the main carer herself has LD, she may find the complexities of the professional network too daunting to deal with, or may have difficulty being articulate and assertive, so may require professional support to achieve the best for her child. For looked-after children, the foster carer or residential social worker may not be able or willing to act as if they had parental responsibility, so the social worker from the child care team or children's disability team may have to take on an advocacy role for the child. If the child is being abused in any way by a carer, then social care may need to exercise its safeguarding role.

Any other involved professional may perceive a need to highlight the child's needs or wishes, and if so, should discuss these first with the child's carers and then if necessary with relevant other professionals. (The carers may be bypassed when there is reason to think that a discussion with them might endanger the child, for instance in cases of severe physical abuse or factitious and induced illness. *See* Chapter 12 on Child Abuse and Safeguarding.)

Liaison

Because children with LD often have a complex combination of problems, there may be professionals of several different disciplines involved. It is important to maintain links between the different services. This may be achieved by: copying letters; telephone calls; informal conversations; or multi-professional meetings. Commonly involved professionals and services include the following.

➤ A *community paediatrician* is likely to have met many children with LD in the Child Development Centre, and often maintains contact. She may take on a coordinating role amongst the different specialist services involved.

➤ A *children's learning disability service*. There is huge variation throughout the UK in how these services are configured across the country. They may for instance be: uni-disciplinary (usually consisting of specialist nurses or psychologists), part of the specialist CAMHS team, separate from the specialist CAMHS team, or non-existent.

➤ *Social care* teams. Depending on local criteria, children with LD may be eligible to have a social worker in the Children's Disability team, but some may require in addition a social worker from the area office, for instance in relation to safeguarding or placement concerns.

➤ *Speech and language therapists* may do direct work with the child, but more commonly work indirectly by setting parents and teachers tasks to help the child improve his skills. They are particularly likely to be involved if the child attends a language unit within a mainstream school, or a special school designated for learning difficulty.

➤ An *educational psychologist* will have to be involved if the child has a statement, and may have done the assessment that revealed the LD. The nature and frequency of ongoing involvement once LD is established varies throughout the UK.

BOX 35.7 Case Example

The health visitor asks the primary mental health worker to meet with four-year-old Lucy and her parents because of increasing concerns about her parents' difficulties in managing Lucy and her six-year-old sister Emily's challenging behaviour.

Lucy was born with profound physical and learning disabilities. She is immobile and has very little recognisable speech. Since the age of two years, Lucy has been banging her head when distressed and screaming whenever she is left alone. Lucy will also wake several times during the night: her mother can get her back to sleep only by holding and rocking her.

Emily – although of apparently normal intelligence – has also developed some behavioural difficulties over the last 12 months. She too has difficulties going to sleep alone and requires her mother or father to stay with her until she falls asleep. She has repeatedly visited Accident and Emergency after inserting objects such as beads up her nose or into her ear canal.

Their parents describe having to supervise both children constantly, with little time for themselves. Lucy's mother is currently on antidepressants and has recently been to see her general practitioner to ask advice about the safety of continuing these in view of her recently discovered pregnancy.

The primary mental health worker, the health visitor and the general practitioner discuss the family at the weekly practice meeting. They realise that several professionals are already involved with the family. They obtain parental consent to hold a professionals meeting, to assess what input has been offered and to coordinate future input. The meeting includes Lucy's community paediatrician, her disability social worker and her community learning disability nurse, who describes the difficulties both parents seem to have in following through with any behavioural interventions. The six professionals wonder whether this might be due to Lucy's mother being reluctant to do anything to cause Lucy distress; they also discuss how much supervision and care Lucy requires, and how her needs are met mainly by her mother. Her father works full-time, and Lucy is in nursery school for afternoons only. The family has previously declined respite care and the offer of a local voluntary organisation to provide some daytime support for Lucy's mother. In view of the current pregnancy, the professionals at the meeting agree that adequate family support is a priority.

The community LD nurse and health visitor agree it would make the most sense for them to take on jointly the lead professional role, with consultation from the primary mental health worker when required. They agree to discuss with Lucy's parents the various options for providing more support, including: changing to full-time nursery school, respite care from social services, involvement of the voluntary organisation, and a sibling support group for Emily.

They emphasise that any parent in such a situation would struggle to meet everyone's needs, particularly in view of the sleep deprivation and the pregnancy. The parents seem to feel heard and understood, and admit they haven't realised that people were trying to help, but thought they were interfering. Once the parents agree to a package involving all four of these options, they move on to discuss which behavioural problem they would like to tackle first. This leads to a detailed management plan being drawn up to help with Lucy's sleep.

Although not all of the two girls' behavioural problems settle immediately, the family has now begun to make better use of the help on offer, and the professional network is more effectively coordinated. All the family start to get enough sleep. Staff at Emily's school are informed of other professionals' concerns: they were not aware there was a problem until they were told of the family's difficulties. Emily stops putting objects into her orifices and her class teacher reports that she has become less withdrawn. Lucy moves to full-time special school just before her baby brother is born. He does not appear to have any developmental difficulties.

REFERRAL

Some children and their families will require referral on to one or more specialist services. If referring to more than one service, it is important to think realistically about how many appointments a family can attend at a given time. It may be better to decide what to do first and what can wait to be addressed at a later time.

Referral may be required to any of the five services mentioned in the previous paragraph, if they are not already involved. For instance, a child with LD who presents with faecal soiling may require referral back to the paediatrician who knows him best, or to a specialist soiling clinic if there is one.

Other specialist services that may be involved include *family therapy* and the *clinical geneticist.* Parents and siblings may have difficulty adjusting to the needs of the young person with LD at particular stages of the life cycle, so may benefit from brief or prolonged family therapy, usually provided by the specialist CAMHS team (*see* Box 35.6 above). Many children may be referred to a clinical geneticist at the time of diagnosis, but siblings may require genetic counselling once they are old enough to understand the implications, for instance, of being a carrier for a genetic disease.

Unfortunately, services for children with LD remain even more variable (throughout the UK) than services for children without LD, so that many children and their families are unable to access an adequate combination of professionals, resulting in unmet need. Individuals with LD are particularly likely to find themselves in a gap without service provision once they have reached 16 or 18 years.

BOX 35.8 Theory points for children with LD

Medical and educational IQ bands have different names.
Causes of mild LD are mainly familial or environmental.
Causes of moderate-to-profound learning disability are mainly genetic or traumatic.
Parents can have major difficulties adjusting to a child with LD: acceptance and adaptation occur at variable rates, and chronic sorrow may require ongoing support.
Effective interventions include social, educational, behavioural and pharmacological.

BOX 35.9 Practice Points for children with LD

Parents may be able to get effective support from the general practitioner, health visitor, children's disability social worker, community LD Nurse, primary mental health worker, CAMHS LD team or other involved professional.
Professional support may need to be ongoing over the child's life span.
There may be a heightened need for such support at times of crisis, such as:
- just after diagnosis
- when the full implications are sinking in
- when behavioural problems seem overwhelming
- when educational needs are not being met
- when the family needs a break to be able to cope
- when formal education is coming to an end
- when parents die.

RESOURCES
Books for young people
- Stern JM, Ben-Ami U, Chesworth M. *Many Ways to Learn: young people's guide to learning disabilities.* Washington DC: Magination Press (American Psychological Association); 1996. This book is written for children aged 8–14 years with learning disabilities: it describes the different kinds of learning disabilities in a non-threatening way and gives practical suggestions about how children can reach their goals.
- Ure J. *Love is Forever.* London: Orchard Books; 2008.
  Thirteen-year-old Tracey knows her love for Paul will last forever. Then one day Paul disappears, taking with him his little sister, Lily. Tracey discovers that Lily is handicapped.

Book for parents
- Holt G, Gratsa A, Bouras N. *Guide to Mental Health for Families and Carers of People with Intellectual Disabilities.* London: Jessica Kingsley; 2004.

Booklet for professionals
- Bernard S, Turk J. *Developing Mental Health Services for Children and Adolescents with Learning Disabilities: a toolkit for clinicians.* London: Royal College of Psychiatrists; 2009. Available at: www.rcpsych.ac.uk/PDF/DevMHservCALDbk.pdf (accessed 3 April 2011).

Websites
- **British Institute of Learning Disability** – A charity committed to improving the quality of life for everyone in the UK with a learning disability: adults and children. The website has information about a variety of helpful publications and lobbying activities. www.bild.org.uk
- **Contact-a-Family** – A UK-wide charity providing advice, information and support to the parents of all disabled children. www.cafamily.org.uk
- **National Autistic Society** – A national charity providing information and advice about autism and autistic spectrum disorders. www.nas.org.uk
- **Royal College of Psychiatrists' Factsheets** – Mental Health and Growing Up, 3rd ed is available at: www.rcpsych.ac.uk
  - **Factsheet 10**: The child with general learning disability: for parents and teachers
  - **Factsheet 11**: Specific learning disabilities: for parents and teachers

REFERENCE
1 Emerson and Hatton. *The Mental Health of Children and Adolescents with Learning Disabilities in Great Britain.* Lancaster: Institute for Health Research, Lancaster University; 2007. Quoted in: *Children and Young People in Mind: the final report of the National CAMHS Review.* London: Department for Children, Schools and Families and Department of Health, UK; 2008. p. 21.

CHAPTER 36

Sleep problems

INTRODUCTION

Preschool

Sleep problems are extremely common in preschool children, and the stress that chronic sleep deprivation may impose on parents can be very distressing and exhausting for parents – who may therefore often ask a professional for help. Some sleep problems, if due to temporary circumstances, settle without intervention. However, if the sleep difficulty has been going on for some time, it is less likely to resolve without some parental intervention. Parents have an important role in helping their children develop good sleep habits.

The pattern of infant sleep differs from that of adults, with more than one sleep-wake cycle occurring in each 24-hour period. This adapts over the first two years to something between eight and 12 hours' night sleep plus an afternoon nap, which is then gradually dropped. As with adults, there is wide variation in sleep requirements.

As growth hormone is released during sleep, adequate sleep is necessary for growth, to restore tired muscles, memory and concentration and to allow the brain to make sense of the day's events and process emotions. Lack of sleep can cause hyperactivity and challenging behaviour.

The basic structure of sleep, including rapid-eye-movement phases (shallow sleep) and non-rapid-eye-movement phases of varying depths, is established in the first year. Children dream extensively during rapid-eye-movement sleep: nightmares are common in primary school children. It is important for parents to understand that all small children wake during the night, but usually settle themselves back to sleep, although parents may be unaware that they have done so. Children who are unable to settle themselves will cry and disturb their parents so are known as night-wakers. If a child has not learnt to settle on his own at bedtime, he may have more difficulty getting back to sleep on his own when he wakes in the night.

BOX 36.1 Case Example

> Single parent Jessica approaches her health visitor about her three-year-old son, Charlie, who is failing to sleep through the night, waking often and calling out to her. This has led to Jessica feeling very sleep-deprived herself – she thinks she is not managing the situation well.

Middle childhood and adolescence

A range of factors may lead to this being a problem also in older children, which may lead to daytime irritability or poor concentration. The amount of sleep varies greatly between individuals (children with ADHD, for instance, appear to require less sleep). Average requirements follow the curve of the growth chart, so that adolescents require more sleep than latency (preadolescent) children, as they grow quicker.

Some important contributing factors to children's sleep impairment may be relevant both for school-age children and for preschoolers:

➤ lack of clear bedtime routines
➤ insufficient exercise during the day
➤ being 'hyped up' by exciting evening activities
➤ stimulation from screens in the bedroom: television, computer or games console
➤ exposure to age-inappropriate material or frightening stories on television, DVD or Internet (including the news and children's cartoons)
➤ real-life traumatic experiences such as domestic violence or sexual abuse
➤ any cause of post-traumatic stress disorder
➤ bad dreams, possibly due to one of the last three
➤ separation anxiety; this is often related to insecure attachment, and so is particularly common for instance in children who have experienced prematurity, parental neglect or family upheaval
➤ overcrowding
➤ poor housing (damp, cold, inadequate ventilation, heat . . .)
➤ noisy neighbours or nearby nightclubs
➤ a bedroom that is unpleasant for some reason (including the last three)
➤ having a difficult temperament, with poorly established circadian rhythms
➤ being allowed to sleep too late in the morning or too long in the afternoon, so that the sleep-wake cycle becomes out of phase with parents'.

BOX 36.2 Case Example

Freddie, aged seven years, is referred to the primary mental health worker by his community school nurse because he has not been concentrating in school. The history she obtains does not sound typical of ADHD: Freddie is lethargic during the day and tends to fall asleep in class. He says he has difficulty going to sleep at night, so she asks about how much exercise he is taking.

It emerges that Freddie has not done any physical education lessons in school for a term-and-a-half because of an ingrown toenail and complications with its treatment. He used to enjoy swimming, but this too has had to stop. Even walking is a bit uncomfortable for him. Asking what sort of exercise Freddie can do, and what he enjoys, reveals that his toe does not bother him while he is cycling, so his parents agree to encourage him to cycle more after school and at weekends.

Their discussion also reveals that Freddie wakes late so has been rushing his breakfast, eating a slice of toast and jam as he hurries out of the door. He agrees to try to get up earlier so as to have a bowl of cereal (sitting down) before he leaves for school. His mother has noticed that he has been leaving the sandwiches in his lunch box and eating only the crisps and chocolate bar. Freddie explains that this is because he likes playing with his friends so much that he wants to finish his lunch as quickly as possible. Freddie's parents explain to him that they are beginning to wonder whether part of the reason he is not listening to his teacher, even when he is awake, is that he is not eating the right sort of food for breakfast or lunch. After some tough negotiations, Freddie agrees to try school dinners for the next half of the term.

The primary mental health worker explores Freddie's bedtime routine. He is good at washing and getting ready for bed, but once he is in bed, he lies awake for a long time before getting off to sleep. Freddie's father used to read him a bedtime story but has recently become busier at work, so he gets home too late. Freddie says that he really used to like his bedtime stories, which helped him to relax. Freddie's father gives in to their combined pressure, and agrees to make an effort to come home in time to read Freddie a story, on condition that his wife allows him to catch up on his e-mails after their evening meal.

When the primary mental health worker reviews the situation the following school term, Freddie's mother says that the combination of all these changes has helped Freddie sleep better and be much more alert in class; his class teacher subsequently confirms this. Freddie's ingrown toenail is now completely better, and he has been able to engage in a range of different forms of exercise.

Sleep problems in older children and adolescents can be related to ***anxiety*** or ***depression***. A good general assessment of how the teenager is functioning in all areas of his life is therefore important. Difficulty getting to sleep, despite going to bed at a reasonable time, may be related more specifically to depression, particularly if it is combined with repeated waking in the middle of the night with difficulty getting back to sleep. General anxiety may delay sleep onset; or there may be specific anxieties about getting to sleep. Examples of family factors are mentioned above: the fear of repeated sexual abuse, or wishing to protect mother from violence by father. Other examples include: a life-threatening illness in one parent, such as cancer or asthma; or the death of one parent engendering a fear that the other will die. Other conditions associated with sleeping difficulties include the afore-mentioned post-traumatic stress disorder and ADHD. Insomnia may also be caused by drugs, occasionally prescribed (for instance salbutamol) or more often bought from friends (such as amphetamine). Alcohol use impairs sleep throughout the night. Excessive use of caffeine-filled drinks may delay sleep onset.

Some adolescents develop a sleep pattern characterised by nocturnal waking: they go to bed in the early hours of the morning and then have difficulty getting up when adults are around. Many teenagers seem to need more sleep than they can easily get, and prefer being awake at night to bothering with mornings. They seem to be geared to a 25-hour day, so gradually become nocturnal if left to their own devices. This can be a problem when it impacts school attendance or getting to work.

BOX 36.3 Case Example

Jeremy, aged 16, has got into the habit of using his computer until 3 or 4 am, then having difficulty waking for college. He tries to catch up at weekends by sleeping on Saturdays and Sundays until well into the afternoon.

The college pastoral support teacher hears about this at a parents' evening. He suggests to Jeremy and his parents that he should 'walk forward' his sleep times even though this seems contrary to common sense, as it is easier to do this than trying to make the times gradually earlier. Jeremy agrees that he will wait until half-term, then postpone his bedtime by two hours each day: after nine days, his bedtime should be 10 pm.

Jeremy's parents are concerned that he won't be able to keep to the 10 pm time, but this will drift forwards again. They get Jeremy to agree that, on nights before a college day, he will turn off his computer by 10 pm and be in bed by 11 pm.

Jeremy has some difficulties with this, but reluctantly agrees to it, on the basis that he enjoys his college course more when he is not falling asleep. He manages to get to sleep usually between 11 pm and midnight on nights when it matters, but makes the most of Friday and Saturday nights to stay up late.

Parents

It is not just children who suffer from impaired sleep: parents and siblings are also affected if one child disturbs the rest of the family repeatedly over successive nights. Parents may experience impaired concentration, irritability, worsening relationships (at home or at work), anxiety or low mood. Reluctance of one child to go to sleep in the evening may make it impossible for a couple to have any together time to themselves, and may prevent siblings from asking friends over.

The leaflet on sleep written specifically for parents referenced under 'Resources' below may be very useful, but might require perseverance for some parents – and so be more effective when accompanied by professional help.

The sort of behavioural measures described in the two case examples in Boxes 36.1 and 36.2 may not work if parents are exhausted and have short tempers. Getting angry with a child who is refusing to go to sleep is likely to keep him awake (perhaps inadvertently reinforcing his behaviour): calmness is required. Sometimes it is necessary to break the cycle of child sleeplessness, leading to parental sleep deprivation, leading to fraught nerves all round: parents may need some sort of break before any management plan is attempted. One way of doing this is to share the nights out so that each parent can catch up on some sleep. Another way is to start a new routine when at least one parent is off work – but the danger of doing this is that the family's routine may not be the same then as usual. A third way is to arrange medication for the child – so that at least the parents can have a rest (*see* below). But in general, behavioural methods are preferable to medication for sleep issues in young children: medication can have side effects and provides only short term relief, whereas a behavioural management programme can provide a long-term solution.

OTHER COMMON SLEEP DISORDERS (PARASOMNIAS)

Nightmares

Dreams and nightmares occur during rapid-eye-movement sleep. It is not clear at what age children start to have nightmares, but it may well be before they are able to talk well enough to describe them. Nightmares definitely occur during the second year of life and are common between three and 10. There are few children who do not have nightmares at some stage, often triggered by something seen on television or experienced during the day. Parents can be reassured that the occasional nightmare is quite normal and not a sign of emotional disturbance.

Children suffering from nightmares will cry out or wake and be obviously frightened. They remember parts of the nightmare and can often describe the dream to their parents, at the time or the next morning. They may be frightened to go back to sleep in case the nightmare recurs.

A clear history of trauma, such as a road traffic accident, makes it easy to understand nightmares. The clinician should consider the possibility of parent-inflicted trauma, such as sexual abuse or domestic violence.

TABLE 36.1 The difference between nightmares, night terrors and sleepwalking

	Nightmares	**Night terrors**	**Sleepwalking**
Timing	Usually in the second half of the night's sleep	Usually in the first third of the night's sleep	Usually in the first third of the night's sleep
Type of sleep	Rapid-eye-movement, shallow sleep	Deep sleep	Deep sleep
Content	Scary or sinister events, remembered or imagined	No conscious memory (but parents sometimes say the terror relates to real, frightening events)	No conscious memory
Management	Help the child talk about the dream, and relate it if appropriate to real events Change the ending	If it occurs at roughly the same sort of time each night, wake the child before this period of deep sleep begins	Keep the child safe: lock outside doors and ensure that windows, if open, could not allow a child to fall through
Significance	Occur sometime to almost everyone May reflect trauma or abuse	Very alarming for parents May perhaps sometimes be a reflection of trauma Do the child no harm	Parents may feel they have to wake up to keep the child safe, although this is usually not necessary, providing the above common-sense precautions are taken

Night terrors

Children with night terrors may also cry out and appear to wake; so how are they different from nightmares? The differences are shown in Table 36.1. Night terrors occur either in deep sleep, or when there is a rapid shift from deep to very light sleep, which can result in an effective overshoot into an extremely aroused state. The child looks as if he is having a terrible experience, often screaming and looking terrified, with eyes wide open. He may be mumbling incoherently. It is not possible to get any account from the child of his experience: if the parents can, then it is more likely to be a nightmare. He appears awake but is not, and will usually fall into a calm sleep after a few minutes if left alone. In contrast to nightmares, the child will have no memory of the episode in the morning.

Night terrors often run in families, and can occur in children of varying ages. They do *not* usually indicate any underlying psychological problem, although the authors have seen them occur in children who are stressed for a variety of reasons – of which parents are usually aware.

BOX 36.4 Case Example

> Nigel begins to have frequent night terrors at the age of 18 months. His mother is convinced these are related to his witnessing some domestic violence before his father left – which was when he was about a year old.

Sleepwalking

Sleepwalking occurs at a similar stage of sleep to night terrors. As with night terrors, the child will have no memory of the event in the morning. It is common, particularly in school age children, and there is often a family history. The relevance of sleep-walking is that it is potentially dangerous, in that a child could fall out of a window or walk into the street – but children never seem to fall down stairs and rarely seem to come to any harm.

ASSESSMENT

As with any behavioural problem, accurate assessment of the situation is essential: asking what happens and when, what comes before (antecedents) and what comes afterwards (consequences).

History of the presenting complaint

What exactly happens? How long has it been going on? What is making it particularly difficult now? Find out exactly which element of the problem is most challenging for each involved parent or caregiver – and what each expects. Are parental expectations realistic? If parents expect a child to go to bed early *and* allow them to sleep in at weekends, they are likely to be disappointed. Does each parent have different expectations?

Family history

There may be relevant changes or losses such as house moves, family separations or domestic violence that may have an effect on the child's sleep. Do siblings affect the index child's sleep, or are they affected by it? For instance, does he share a room?

Developmental and medical history

This may help to explain how some difficulties with sleep have developed. The quality or amount of sleep may be affected by conditions such as the following.

➤ With *eczema*, affected skin may itch a lot during the night.

➤ Nocturnal *asthma* may keep the child awake.

➤ Large tonsils can obstruct the airway and cause a pattern of intermittent sleeping and waking (*sleep apnoea*).

➤ A child who has been very ill, for instance due to *premature* birth, may have parents who are understandably anxious about leaving him to sleep alone. A parent may think, if not act on the impulse: 'I need to wake him up to make sure he's still breathing'.

➤ Prolonged *hospitalisation* can disrupt sleep rhythms, because the child has adjusted to sleeping in a busy, noisy environment that is often well lit, and may be disoriented by returning to the very different home environment.

➤ Children with severe *developmental delay* or brain injuries are more susceptible to sleep disorders.

➤ Children with other developmental difficulties may have specific sleep difficulties. For instance, a child with a visual impairment may need support to organise his body clock; or a child with ADHD may require less sleep than most children of his age.

➤ Children with an autistic spectrum disorder who are sensitive to noise may be kept awake by things that seem quiet to everyone else.

Strategies already tried

Find out what the parents have tried, how they have implemented ideas and how long they have persevered. How long did they try any changes in routine and what effect did it have on the situation? Does each parent have a different way of responding to the situation? Are others involved in generating solutions? Parents may discuss at this time how upset and distressed they and the child can get over this issue.

BOX 36.5 Case Example

The parents of Jemima, aged two years, have tried leaving her in her cot to cry. Although her mother is all for letting her cry until she stops, her father cannot bear to hear this, so he goes at once to comfort her. It appears to the interviewer that Jemima enjoys the cuddles she receives as a result.

Typical day and night routine

It is important to know what happens during the day with regard to other routines and especially around nap times, mealtimes and drinks. There also needs to be a clear picture of the night-time and settling-to-bed routine.

At this stage, it may be possible to formulate the problem and give simple advice. If not, the next stage is to establish the sleep pattern. The best way to build up an accurate picture of this is to ask one of the parents to keep a sleep diary for a week. A typical example is shown in Table 36.2. The diary can also include extra information such as which parent takes charge or more details about bedtime routines. It is very important to establish that the parent understands exactly how to fill in the diary, and the reasons for its use. Depending on the information obtained from the diary, it may be possible to suggest practical measures to resolve the problem, or go on to use a specific behavioural programme.

Adolescents

The older the child, the more necessary it is to do a general assessment, as other conditions linked to the sleep difficulty become more likely.

MANAGEMENT
Prevention

It may be worth asking about sleep as part of the assessment of *any* presenting problem. In particular, preschool behaviour problems, school difficulties, ADHD and mood disorders may all be closely linked to sleep disorders. If a sleep problem is discussed before it has become entrenched, it may respond better to simple advice, such as about the importance of establishing good bedtime routines, or the value of ensuring that young children get used to settling themselves to sleep.

Self-settling

There are various simple measures that will help a child to settle himself to sleep. The younger the child, the easier these are to institute. The aim is for the child to learn to fall asleep on his own, and the parent's role is to help him learn how to do this.

The first step is usually to establish a **regular routine**, which most children thrive on. This can start with daytime and then progress to the evening and bedtime. Wake your child at the same time each morning; this gets the day off to a regular start. It may be necessary initially to move any daytime naps to before 2 pm, in order to give the child a better chance of settling at a reasonable time in the evening. Routine becomes more important as bedtime approaches. Most children need a wind-down time before bed to help them sleep well at night. The same thing needs to happen in the same order every night for a bedtime routine to be successful.

The following may contribute to the success of a **bedtime ritual** – a fixed progression of events leading up to bedtime, which can help a small child tell bedtime is getting close, and an older child wind down. The idea is that the child will be relaxed enough on getting into bed at least to lie quietly, if not go to sleep.

TABLE 36.2 Example of a sleep diary

Day and date	What time did the child wake up?	Did the child need wakening?	What was the child's mood on waking?	Times and duration of daytime naps	What time did the bedtime routine start?	How did child respond to bedtime routines?	Parents' actions at child's bedtime	What time did the child go to sleep?	Times and duration of night-time waking	Parents' responses to child waking
Monday										
Tuesday										
Wednesday										
Thursday										
Friday										
Saturday										
Sunday										

➤ Ask parents to decide what time they would like the child to be in bed: they can then work backwards to build the structure of the routine.

➤ Regular mealtimes can help build up a routine. The child should reach bedtime neither hungry nor too full. Stimulating drinks and foods should be avoided for about six hours before bedtime – which means anything containing caffeine, including chocolate. High-fat foods may impair sleep quality. Sugary snacks are probably not a good idea just before bedtime, not only because of the effect on teeth, but also because they can make some children more energetic. So any pre-bedtime snacks should ideally be low in fat and sugar.

➤ Drinking enough fluids will keep the child adequately hydrated and may aid sleep. A hot milky drink may be a valuable part of the bedtime routine. A child may learn that saying he is thirsty is a way of postponing sleep-time and getting adult attention, so it is important to set advance limits on how many drinks are allowed. It may be important to remind the child to empty his bladder just before going to bed – so he doesn't have to wake up for this.

➤ Watching television, playing computer games or using the Internet too close to bedtime may be too stimulating for some children. Alternative activities may need to be promoted, such as playing with a doll's house or models, drawing or colouring in, doing jigsaw puzzles or playing with Duplo or Lego or other construction kit.

➤ There should be a ritual around cleaning teeth and washing or having a bath. Once the child accepts this, it should be predictable and relaxing.

➤ The bedroom should be quiet, comfortable and conducive to sleep, for instance with a night light, fresh air, child-friendly decorations and an appropriate temperature. The room should be dark(-ish) even if it is daylight outside (such as in midsummer) – so curtains need to be thick enough. Younger children may feel more secure with a favourite soft toy or blanket, which should remain close while they are asleep. Are there any potentially frightening things on the walls or cupboards or ceiling? It may be better to keep distractions such as toys and television in another room if possible.

➤ Reading a bedtime story can help a child relax, unwind and feel secure. Set a reasonable limit on how long you are going to read for, depending on the child's age. Story or lullaby compact discs or tapes can be used, but may not be quite so reassuring and comforting, particularly for a younger or insecure child. Playing a particular piece of relaxing music may also be reassuring, but some children may be upset if the music is not playing when they wake up in the middle of the night. Similarly, if parents insist on using a television as a comforter, and leave it on until the child falls asleep, he may be distressed by finding it is off when he wakes up.

➤ Children are also comforted and relaxed by cuddles and kisses, but these should not be repeated endlessly. Some children may demand repeated reassurance of this sort as a tactic to prolong bedtime.

➤ Any bedtime routine needs to be used consistently from night to night, by any parent who lives at home and by any other adults who care for the child, such as a grandparent or non-resident parent.

Once the child is asleep, it is important to ensure he stays that way, or at least goes back to sleep readily when he wakes up. Check that parents have made sure that any night light is not too bright and that there are no noises near his bedroom to wake him up. Advise parents that if he does wake up, they should engage in no more than minimal comforting conversation. If the child asks frequently for drinks during the night, for instance of milk, a parent should try to phase these out gradually as the child gets older.

BOX 36.6 Case Example

Sharon, the mother of three-year-old Karl, approaches her health visitor about his sleep routine: she is concerned that he will not settle when she puts him to bed and then wakes frequently throughout the night.

The history reveals that Karl's parents separated 18 months ago, leading to a house move, after which he initially spent most nights in Sharon's bed. He no longer wants to sleep in his own room. Karl has a good daytime routine, but does not have a regular bedtime – Sharon puts him in her bed when he feels tired or lets him fall asleep in front of the television on the sofa, and then carries him to his own bed. He then moves to her bed the first time in the night that he wakes.

The health visitor explains to Sharon that, in order to begin a regular sleep routine, Karl needs to learn to fall asleep in his own bed. They agree a clear bedtime routine for Karl including a bath, after which he should stay upstairs, followed by a warm drink and then a bedtime story in his own bed. They also agree that Sharon will explain this new routine to Karl and set up a reward chart with a sticker for each night he spends in his bed. Sharon decides she will use a gradual rather than a sudden programme for settling Karl: initially, she will sit by his bed until he settles, then over the next few weeks move to a chair by the door and then into the hallway. The health visitor warns Sharon that Karl is likely to be quite upset to start with about these changes, so she will need to be sure to give him extra support. She arranges to telephone Sharon regularly over the next few weeks.

With this telephone support, and the option to phone at other times if necessary, Sharon sticks to the new routine. Karl learns to settle in his own bed again. He adapts to the regular bedtime, and his night-waking decreases – but when he does wake in the night, Sharon returns him to his bed and settles him there, using the same graded approach. After six weeks, Karl has a satisfactory sleep routine, and there is no more need for his sticker chart.

Behavioural interventions

If this basic approach of establishing a bedtime routine and a restful setting for sleep is insufficient, then further measures will be needed. Once parents have had an opportunity to catch up on their own sleep, there are two different approaches to consider: *gradual management* and *leaving the child to cry*.

Gradual management (controlled crying)

This technique is more acceptable to many parents than leaving their child to scream for long periods. It may take slightly longer to work but is just as effective, and often less traumatic.

Many parents will say they have tried controlled crying before and it did not work. Closer questioning usually reveals that they could not stand the screaming and gave up too soon. *It is vital to stress to parents before they start this technique that the screaming will get worse before it gets better, and that they should not give up in the middle of the treatment programme, as this sends the child the message that if he screams for long enough the parents will give in.* Both parents must agree to using this technique, doing it properly and supporting each other. It is worth advising parents to warn neighbours so they are not anxious about their reaction. Parents must *explain to the child* what is going to happen.

➤ A parent settles the child briefly, *stopping short of him falling asleep,* and leaves the room. The bedroom door is left ajar.

➤ She does not return for five minutes unless the child gets out of bed, in which case she returns to him and tells him that she will shut the bedroom door if he gets out of bed again.

➤ At five minutes, she returns to the child and settles him briefly (for about two minutes) and then leaves the room again. *She must leave the room before he falls asleep.*

➤ Ten minutes later, she returns and settles him briefly again.

➤ Fifteen minutes later, she visits the child again and subsequently visits at 15 minute intervals until the child is asleep. She must always leave the room before the child falls asleep since the object of the exercise is to help him learn how to fall asleep on his own. All she has to do is quieten him.

➤ After the first night, the intervals are increased by 5 minutes, that is 10 minutes to the first settle, then 15, and then 20 (*see* Table 36.3).

➤ Most children will be settling well by the end of a week. Nearly always, the problem has resolved before getting to 45-minute timings.

TABLE 36.3 Helping a child fall asleep alone: a graded approach
How long to wait before entering the child's room to comfort him (in minutes):

Day	First time	Second time	Third and subsequent times
1	5	10	15
2	10	15	20
3	15	20	25
4	20	25	30
5	25	30	35
6	30	35	40
7	35	40	45

Sometimes, the situation deteriorates to such an extent that the child is entirely unable to settle alone, and the parent is spending enormous amounts of time in the child's room, often sitting or lying by the cot or holding him until he falls asleep. In these cases, the aim is for *very gradual change*. The parents must gradually encourage the child to sleep alone. Initially the child lies in the cot or bed with a parent just touching. Over several evenings, the parent slowly moves away, first sitting on a chair by the bed, then moving the chair gradually nearer the door, until eventually she is outside. The parent should be encouraged to have something to do other than paying the child attention, such as reading, knitting or listening to music. If the parent has been singing to the child for hours, then encourage her to hum more and more softly each evening.

Letting the child cry

This is quick and very successful if the parents can manage it, but many parents find it too stressful. As with the previous approach, both parents should agree about the details of the technique, should have prepared a suitable environment and should have warned the neighbours. Parents *must explain to the child* what is going to happen: once he has been kissed goodnight, he should lie quietly in his bed and wait until he falls asleep, as they are not going to come in to him when he cries.

➤ The child should not be able to get out of the door but should be able to reassure himself that the parents are still around and have not deserted him.

➤ The parents need to let the child know that they are still around by carrying on normal routines such as having the television on or chatting together. This is in contrast to the usual parental practice of creeping around silently 'to let him get to sleep'.

➤ The parents must have something to do besides listening to the screams or they will not be able to stand it.

➤ The total duration of crying before sleep should be recorded on a chart.

➤ If the child vomits or rips off his nappy as a result of crying, he should be cleaned up with the minimum of fuss and no chat and returned to bed.

➤ Both parents must understand the *crying gets worse before it subsides*. This is an example of the **extinction burst**: any behaviour that succeeds in attracting attention, or that is encouraged by social reinforcement, will initially intensify if attention is withdrawn. If parents can last out for the first four nights, the crying will then gradually subside. The record kept will show this more clearly than the recollections of a fraught and somewhat guilty parent.

➤ Next morning the child can be praised for going to sleep on his own, and given a reward if a reward system has been set up.

For the child who repeatedly comes out of his bedroom once well settled, a physical barrier such as a stair-gate in the doorway is a useful ploy. This can keep him in his room without him feeling closed in. If this is not practical, the child should be firmly and silently returned to his room.

With either of these two approaches, it is important to praise the child as much as possible for any small success. Parents should remain positive; getting into an argument or being critical may simply postpone settling time. *See* Chapter 13 on Behaviour Management for more detail about how to use praise. Hugs may also help.

Reward systems

Added to either gradual management or leaving the child to cry, a reward system may improve success: breaking tasks down into small steps and rewarding each step. For instance, the first step might be coming no further than the top of the stairs; the next step might be coming no further than the bedroom doorway; and the next might be staying quiet. The aim is to have the child lying quietly in bed, ready for sleep. This is usually more realistic than setting as a target a particular time of sleep onset.

Reward systems can be used in a number of other ways, especially for children over three years old. A chart for stars or stickers or smiley faces can be used, or a string next to the bed to hold beads. A reward should be given as soon as possible after completing a set task. Examples include (in order of difficulty): getting into bed without fuss, staying quietly in bed for at least three minutes while mother goes downstairs, and staying quietly in bed for 10 minutes. Once a behaviour has been established for a week, a new task is set and the colour or nature of the reward is changed.

Night waking

This is really a failure to settle back to sleep after ordinary waking at night. Approximately half of night wakers will be found to have a problem settling to sleep in the evening when a careful history is taken. In these cases, the settling problem should be dealt with first and this may solve the night-time problem.

Often this problem arises because the falling-to-sleep routine involves a cue that is missing in the middle of the night when the child awakens, such as a story-tape, music or the television. It is therefore worth working on removing these distractions when first settling in order to help the child stay settled later on. If he falls asleep easily in the evening when there is light from the landing, but finds it hard to settle when he wakes at night and it is dark and silent, it may be worth trying to duplicate these conditions at night by leaving the landing light on.

The initial approach is to attempt to settle the child, leaving the room before he falls asleep, or firmly return him to bed if he is coming into the parents' room. If this fails, then a graded approach, as already described for settling to sleep, should be used. It is worth remembering that it is much harder to leave a child to scream in the middle of the night, and it is even more important to have warned the neighbours.

Older children and adolescents

Once habits are firmly formed, they may be more difficult to change. So sleep management in older children is more challenging than in preschoolers. Table 36.4 provides a summary of some useful tips for improving sleep hygiene. It is addressed to the child, so could be printed off for older children or adolescents; parents can translate it into what it implies they can do to help. For instance, reading a book in bed should be translated for a younger child into an adult reading a story to the

TABLE 36.4 Suggestions for improving sleep hygiene

	Things that will help you get sleepy	Things that may keep you awake	Things that will help your bedtime routine	Things that will help you stay asleep
Diet	Is the time of your latest meal best to enable you to get to sleep?	Any caffeine-containing drinks or foods can keep you awake – including chocolate Alcohol can make you wake up a lot	Try a warm, milky drink before going to bed If you have a snack before bedtime, make it low sugar and low fat, such as an apple, a carrot, banana or dry toast	Not being hungry or too full
Exercise	Have enough exercise during the day Have some mild exercise before your bedtime routine starts	Not having any exercise	Do something physically active between school and bedtime	Being physically tired
Body clock	Make the room dark enough – use thick enough curtains to prevent light coming in	Having naps during the day	Wind down gradually in the evening Have a regular bedtime routine that starts about 15 minutes before you go to bed	Go back to sleep if you wake up too early Get up early enough in the morning to feel tired by bedtime the next night
Emotional	Review the day before you go to sleep – by yourself or with someone else Have a cuddle with someone if possible	Having an argument or experiencing some upset just before bedtime	Do calming things just before getting into bed Once in bed, relaxing activities may help – listening to music or a story, reading a book . . .	An emotionally calm atmosphere in the household
Psychological	Get things ready for the next day before you start your bedtime routine	Watching television in bed	Turn off screen machines about half an hour before bedtime Imagine a relaxing scene as you lie down	Write down nightmares if you have them Don't stay out of bed more than you have to in the middle of the night
Physical	Have a warm bath	Bedding falling off so that you get cold: make sure it will stay on you	Taking slow, deep breaths as you lie down	Is your bed comfortable? Do you have a comfortable pillow and fresh bedding?
Environmental	Make sure your bedroom is as free of clutter as possible	Noise from inside or outside the home	Make sure your bedroom is a relaxing setting	Make sure the bedroom is the right temperature – usually 16–20°C Are there any draughts?

child. The astute reader will notice that the content is similar to the list of bullet points in the self-settling section above.

For young people who lie awake for ages, or wake up and cannot get back to sleep, an additional practical tip may help, which is too detailed to fit in the table:

> If you find you are wide awake for so long that you are getting wound up, get out of bed and do something relaxing for 15-20 minutes. Then repeat your bedtime routine and go back to bed. If you are wide awake but feel calm, try to stay in bed and fill your mind with something relaxing, while taking slow, deep breaths. For instance, if you find beaches relaxing, imagine in detail taking a gentle stroll along a beach, and enjoying the sound of the waves. Imagine lying in the sunshine and feeling the warmth of the sun on your skin. Elaborate your image as necessary: it may soon turn into a dream . . .

It is probably worth re-emphasising that sleep problems in adolescents may indicate other problems, such as anxiety, depression, ADHD or post-traumatic stress disorder, so adequate assessment is necessary before giving any advice about sleep hygiene.

Management of parasomnias (nightmares, night terrors and sleepwalking)

For *nightmares*, a parent should go quickly to the child, then hold and reassure him until he slips back to sleep: note that this is the *opposite* of the gradual withdrawal recommended above. Providing a night light or a comforting toy may also help.

As nightmares often occur at a time in a child's development when he is questioning the world around him, it may be worth checking if the child is asking questions about death or other potentially worrying topics, and providing explanations that he can understand. If nightmares occur frequently, or if there is a recurring theme, encourage parents to explore their child's fears. These may be related to real-life dilemmas or scary situations – with which the child may need adult help, but does not know how to ask. Drawing pictures or playing imaginative games may be easier for him than talking. If a nightmare is repeated, a parent may be able to guide the child through altering the end of the dream, such as facing and scaring away the monster.

For *night terrors*, first reassure parents by giving accurate information, and explaining that children will grow out of this behaviour. Night terrors are frightening to watch, and parents need to be told that the child is asleep and will come to no harm. Parents should be advised not to try to wake the child.

If the night terrors are occurring frequently, they can be very disruptive to the family. In these cases, *anticipatory waking* can be used, and will be most effective if they occur at roughly the same time each night. The child is woken about half an hour before the expected onset, and allowed to go back to sleep after a few minutes. This changes the pattern of the sleep stages, and often has the effect of abolishing the problem, sometimes after as little as one week.

For *sleepwalking*, information for parents is again helpful, but reassurance is inappropriate, because a child could come to harm, as parents are usually well aware. They need to ensure the child's safety by checking that the child cannot fall out of a bedroom window or get through an outside door. During the sleepwalking episode, the child should be gently steered back to bed, and the whole episode played down. Anticipatory waking can be tried if the problem is frequent.

Medication

Medication is occasionally prescribed in younger children as a short-term measure when parents are thoroughly exhausted. Carers may have difficulty persuading their general practitioner that this is appropriate, in view of the high success rate of behavioural treatments.

Some older children have developed a bedtime routine that parents may find difficult or be unwilling to shift. If these children have a predisposing condition, most commonly ADHD or another recognised developmental problem, they may benefit from longer-term use of medication to make it easier to get off to sleep.

At the time of writing this chapter, the medication most commonly used for these indications by paediatricians and child psychiatrists is *melatonin*. This is probably because it is a naturally occurring hormone and it seems to have few side effects. The dose required may be greater for younger than older children: a starting dose is usually 2 mg, but this can be gradually increased – if there is no response – up to 20 mg. Side effects are uncommon with this approach, but may include headache, dizziness, nausea, restlessness, itching or an increased heart rate. Unfortunately for sleepless children and their parents, melatonin is not yet licensed in the UK below the age of 55 years, which makes many general practitioners reluctant to prescribe it. This is not necessarily a problem, as many such children are already under the care of a specialist.

REFERRAL

Many health centres or consortia of health visitors have set up sleep clinics for preschool children, which have a high degree of success. So in general, referral at this age should not be necessary unless there are complicating issues such as developmental delay or attachment difficulties (as is likely in fostered or adopted children) – in which case it may be worthwhile to refer to a community paediatrician or a dedicated Looked after Children CAMHS team. In some areas, involving a primary mental health worker may be more appropriate. For older children with sleep difficulties, the need for referral is likely to be determined chiefly by the nature of any associated problems.

BOX 36.7 Practice Points for sleep management

Assessment is important: this can include a careful history and a sleep diary.
Failure to settle should be tackled before night waking.
Behavioural methods work very well for both these problems in small children.
Night terrors (and sometimes sleepwalking) can be managed by anticipatory waking.
Nocturnal teenagers who want to be able to get up in the morning should move their bedtime forwards rather than backwards.

RESOURCES
Books for children

- Lite L, Fox KC. *The Goodnight Caterpillar: a children's relaxation story to improve sleep, manage stress, anxiety, anger.* London: LiteBooks.net LLC; 2007.
  This colourfully illustrated book uses guided imagery to help children settle to sleep.
- Lite L. *Boy and a Bear.* London: Partners Publishing Group; 2001.
  This book uses breathing exercises to help children relax during the day or at night.
- Mayle P. *Sweet Dreams and Monsters: beginner's guide to dreams and nightmares and things that go bump under the bed.* London: Macmillan Children's Books; 1987.
  This is a fun book for younger children discussing dreams and nightmares.
- Waddell M, Firth B. *Can't You Sleep, Little Bear?* London: Walker Books; 2005.
  This book for 2–5 year olds won the Kate Greenaway Medal and the Smarties Book Prize.
- Brown MW, Hurd C. *Goodnight, Moon.* London: Macmillan Children's Books; 2010.
  A young bunny rabbit goes through his bedtime routine, bidding goodnight to all of the familiar objects and characters in his room. This story addresses toddlers' fears of the dark and going to bed.

Books for parents

- Department of Education. *Information for Parents: sleep.* London: Department of Education; 2010. Available at: http://publications.dcsf.gov.uk/eOrderingDownload/ES82.pdf (accessed 4 April 2011).
- Ferber R. *Solve your Child's Sleep Problems.* London: Dorling Kindersley; 2006.
  This book is about how to deal with sleep problems in children of different ages.
- Huntley R. *The Sleep Book for Tired Parents: help for solving children's sleep problems.* 3rd ed. London: Souvenir Press; 2004.
  This book covers children from birth to six years and gives a choice of approaches to managing commonly encountered sleep problems.
- Quine L. *Solving Children's Sleep Problems: a step by step guide for parents.* Huntingdon: Beckett Karlson; 1997.
  This comprehensive, step-by-step guide covers the age range from birth to 18 years.
- Stores, G. *Sleep problems in Children and Adolescents (The Facts).* Oxford: Oxford University Press; 2008.

Websites

Scope – This is a charity for children with cerebral palsy, but can help with sleep difficulties also in children who have other types of special need:
- www.scope.org.uk
- www.sleepsolutions.org.uk

CHAPTER 37

Adjustment disorder and post-traumatic stress disorder

INTRODUCTION

Terminology

Whilst the reactions of individuals to traumatic events have been described for years, our ways of understanding this have changed. The term 'post-traumatic stress disorder' (PTSD) evolved from previous descriptions of the problems of *war veterans* such as:

➤ combat neurosis
➤ shell shock – a popular term in the First World War
➤ survivor syndrome.

Gradually, it became generally recognised that a relatively homogeneous *constellation of symptoms* can arise not just from war experiences but also from other traumatic events such as rape, natural disasters such as earthquakes or accidents such as a car crash – in fact anything highly stressful, threatening or catastrophic. Emotional reactions at the time may include overwhelming fear, helplessness or horror. In a minority of those who experience such trauma, there emerges subsequently a characteristic pattern of psychological symptoms that persists, sometimes causing considerable impairment.

Clinical features

The three *core features* of post-traumatic stress disorder in adults are:

➤ *re-experiencing* the traumatic event(s) while asleep in dreams or while awake in flashbacks
➤ *avoidance* of situations, people or things that remind the individual of the traumatic event
➤ *increased arousal*, such as jumpiness, difficulty sleeping or hypersensitivity.

Recognition of a similar pattern of symptoms in children eventually emerged. There are four rather than three groups of symptoms, which must follow exposure to a traumatic event and last for over a month.

Criteria for the diagnosis of post-traumatic stress disorder in childhood have been proposed as follows:[1]

➤ *Re-experiencing* of the event. There must be at least one of:
  — post-traumatic play (compulsively repetitive representations of parts of the trauma)
  — re-enactment of some traumatic experiences through play
  — other recurrent recollections, such as repeatedly intrusive memories or flashbacks (in any sensory modality)
  — nightmares
  — flashbacks
  — dissociation
  — distress at exposure to reminders of the event.
➤ *Numbing of responsiveness*. There must be at least one of:
  — constriction of play
  — social withdrawal
  — restricted range of affect
  — loss of acquired developmental skills, especially language regression and loss of toilet training.
➤ *Increased arousal*. There must be at least one of:
  — night terrors
  — difficulty going to sleep other than due to fear of nightmares or of the dark
  — night waking not related to nightmares or night terrors.
➤ *New fears or aggression*. There must be at least one of:
  — new aggression
  — new separation anxiety
  — fear of toileting alone
  — fear of the dark
  — any other new fears of things or situations not obviously related to the trauma.

BOX 37.1 Case Example

Andrea, aged three years, was sitting in the back seat of the family car on a routine Tuesday while her mother drove her to nursery school. Another car emerged from a side road without seeing their car, and collided with Andrea's side, fortunately hitting mainly the front half.

Andrea was carefully buckled into her seat-belt, so she suffered no more than minor bruises, although the car was damaged beyond repair. Her mother was physically unharmed.

For several months after the accident, Andrea suffers disturbed sleep, and insists on spending the entire night in her parents' bed. It is not clear whether she is having nightmares, but she cannot recall any dreams. She becomes more clingy than her younger brother Henry, two years her junior. She is reluctant to leave the house or play with friends. She flinches whenever she hears a car breaking. She cries if her mother drives the same route to nursery school as on the unfortunate Tuesday, but is quiet if they travel on an alternative route. Her behaviour becomes more difficult to control, and she shows aggression towards Henry for the first time.

These symptoms gradually subside over the course of a year.

The above definition has the advantage of applying to **pre-verbal children**, who appear to have non-verbal, post-traumatic memories that significantly affect behaviour and psychosocial development and which may be retained for a significant period.[2,3] Infants and young children may demonstrate re-experiencing through post-traumatic play and trauma re-enactment.[4]

BOX 37.2 Case Example

> Zelda is seven years old when her foster mother takes her to specialist CAMHS because her behaviour is so difficult to manage. During the assessment, Zelda approaches the doll's house, finds some figures there, and puts them in sexual postures with each other.
>
> Although the past history from social services is rather complicated, it seems that Zelda's mother had serious mental health problems, and probably allowed Zelda to be sexually abused by a number of unidentified males. The assessing CAMHS workers conclude that she is re-enacting some of the trauma she witnessed or experienced.

Children may initially present with disorganised and agitated behaviour, rather than fear, hopelessness or horror. The way the subsequent symptoms evolve can vary greatly, not only because traumatic events differ in their nature and because age plays a large part, but also because of individual differences in temperament, resilience and the way emotions are expressed.

A key determinant of the pattern of presentation is developmental stage (*see* Table 37.1). According to Piaget,[5] a young child at the preoperational stage of cognitive development is dominated by her egocentrism, or tendency to view the world from her own perspective. Therefore she is very likely to see her role in any (traumatic) event as central – and may even feel partially responsible for what has happened. In middle childhood and adolescence, making comparisons with others is important in the development of self-esteem and fashioning a self-image. Traumatic life events may lead not only to post-traumatic stress disorder, but also via negative self-appraisal to depression[6] – or something intermediate between the two (*see* the section below on 'Adjustment disorder' and the case example in Box 37.6).

Additional features that may occur specifically in childhood which are not mentioned in the bullet points above include the following.[7,8]

➤ An *exaggerated startle response* – This is part of the increased arousal. The startle response is based on a reflex that begins to come under conscious control only during middle childhood. This means that younger children may be less able to manage the emotions associated with arousal, and more likely to feel overwhelmed by them.

➤ *Reduced concentration* – This is part of the numbing of responsiveness and may lead to a decline in academic performance.

➤ *Patchy or confused memory* for the traumatic events – In particular, '*time skew*' describes a child getting muddled about the sequence of trauma-related events when recalling the memory.

TABLE 37.1 Presentation of PTSD at different ages

Developmental stage of child	Ways in which PTSD can present
Preschool	Repeated themes in play and behaviour
	Restricted play
	Loss of previously acquired skill
	Night terrors
	Toileting problems
	Development of new fears
School age	Re-enactment in play and drawings
	Time skew or patchy recall of the trauma
	Omen formation
Adolescence	Adult-like symptoms
	Dissociation
	Self-harm
	Aggression
	Alcohol and substance misuse
Any age	Sleep disturbance
	Irritability
	Poor concentration
	Decreased academic performance at school
	Somatic complaints
	Separation anxiety
	Fears
	Avoidance
	Exaggerated startle response

➤ Children may want to make sense of their experiences, sometimes using explanations which make less sense to adults – such as feeling responsible for the traumatic event. Another example of this is '*omen formation*', which is a belief that there were warning signs that predicted the trauma. This can be reassuring for the child, who may believe that, if she is alert enough, she will recognise these warning signs (omens) and so avoid future traumas.

➤ *Somatic complaints* of any sort.[9]

➤ *Irritability* is a common consequence of increased arousal, and may be exacerbated by poor sleep, which can be impaired for a number of reasons.

➤ An important symptom of post-traumatic stress disorder in some young people is **dissociation**. This is a useful mechanism of self-protection that involves *not* remembering the awful things that have happened, or acting as if they have happened to somebody else. It is not generally a conscious process, but children can resort to it after any trauma, particularly sexual abuse. Adolescents are particularly likely to show dissociative features, especially those who have had prolonged or repeated exposure to trauma: presenting features may include self-harm, aggression[10] or substance misuse,[11] which could be seen as a way of attempting to deal with unwanted memories. The habit of dissociating can then contribute to the development of dissociative disorders and borderline personality disorder. Although these labels are more appropriately reserved for adults rather than being applied to under-18s, it is sometimes possible to observe the patterns they describe emerging in adolescents. A more in-depth discussion of these disorders is beyond the scope of this book.

BOX 37.3 Case Example

> After her fifth overdose at the age of 15 years, Nasreen discloses to her family therapist that the man her mother cohabited with after her father left home was not only violent to her mother (already discussed) but also violent to Nasreen, including sexually. Nasreen's mother was not aware of this, and both were in tears as a result of this revelation – which helped to explain to the therapist and her colleagues Nasreen's pattern of repeated self-harm.

BOX 37.4 Case Example

> Olivia, aged 13 years, is in the care of social services due to a complex pattern of abuse and neglect in her family of origin. She is regularly overcome by uncontrollable rages, which have contributed to her moving from one foster placement to another. Her current foster mother has observed her, during some of these rages, talking about herself in the third person, saying for instance: 'She's at it again . . .'
>
> Olivia's therapist in the Looked-After Children's Team looks through the past file. There is no definite evidence that Olivia was sexually abused, but several other family members are convinced this has happened, probably when Olivia was less than five years old.
>
> The therapist asks Olivia whether she remembers anyone sexually abusing her, and Olivia says she does not, but doesn't seem very sure about it. The therapist says she thinks sexual (or other forms of) abuse might have occurred when Olivia was too young to remember: the relevance of this could be that it is contributing to her rages. The rages feel like it is someone else that is getting angry, because it felt like it was someone else getting abused. The therapist says that children who are abused often deal with this by pretending that it is happening to someone else. She asks Olivia whether this idea makes any sense in relation to her rages, and Olivia says it does.

Risk factors: who develops post-traumatic stress disorder?

Whilst anyone can develop post-traumatic stress disorder, girls appear in general to be more susceptible than boys; and less-able children are likely to be more badly affected than those with a greater capacity to understand and explain. These differences seem independent of age and apply to both acute and chronic post-traumatic stress disorder. Experiencing the death or severe injury of a parent at the same time increases the risk to the child.[12] The type of trauma is also important: the proportion of those exposed to a particular trauma who develop post-traumatic symptoms as a consequence is determined to a considerable extent by the nature of the event. As an example, a study of road traffic accidents found that children or adolescents who are passengers in a car accident appear more likely (72%) to develop significant post-traumatic stress disorder symptoms after six weeks than those riding a bicycle or who are pedestrians at the time (30%).[13] It seems that the level of exposure to personal danger correlates with the subsequent severity of symptoms.[14]

Adjustment disorder and other responses to trauma and stress

Most traumatic or stressful events are followed by an understandable emotional reaction, which is usually short-lived and can resolve without any specific intervention. A term such as *'acute stress reaction'* may be used to describe such self-limiting human experiences. Some of those exposed to a traumatic event may develop a longer or more impairing response than this, without the core features of post-traumatic stress disorder, which may be described as an *adjustment disorder*. This range of reactions (*see* Figure 37.1) can be seen as in many ways similar to those following bereavement (*see* Chapter 10): despite much individual variation, identifiable feelings are usually experienced in a certain order, but it is impossible to predict for an individual how long her feelings will last. When symptoms persist or are particularly distressing, or when an individual appears to 'get stuck', the reaction may be considered impairing and the person may require some help to facilitate her adjustment. Some children develop some of the symptoms of post-traumatic stress disorder, but not quite enough for a strict diagnosis, so may be described as having *post-traumatic symptoms*.

The characteristics of *adjustment disorder* are as follows, differentiating it from an acute stress reaction and from post-traumatic stress disorder.

➤ The trauma or psychosocial stressor is usually a relatively mundane event, and at any rate *not* catastrophic. Common examples may include:
 — a house move
 — a school move (particularly when others are *not* moving school)
 — the departure of a best friend
 — the break-up of a relationship – this is especially salient for adolescents
 — the departure of a parent
 — an episode of bullying, particularly one resulting in physical injury or fears for personal safety.

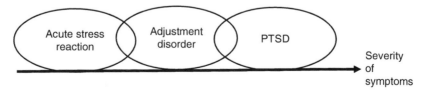

FIGURE 37.1 Responses to trauma or stressful life events

➤ It is *not* a bereavement.

➤ The symptoms generally begin within three months of the precipitating event and generally resolve within six months, but these **time limits** are arbitrary, and children do not usually limit their symptoms to textbook definitions.

➤ There is some form of **distress**, with associated **impairment**. The distress usually shows itself in the form of emotional or behavioural symptoms, which may occur in a variety of combinations and severity. Textbooks tend to describe these symptoms as most often being subclinical forms of depression, anxiety or conduct disorder, but in clinical practice the pattern of difficulty is often not so easily categorised. The impairment affects one or more of home life, school life and friendships.

➤ There may be no need for professional intervention, but sometimes it may be helpful for *someone* (a friend, a parent, or a professional) to **listen** to what has happened and **frame** the reaction as quite **understandable** (considering the emotional impact such an event would have on most people). Further opportunities to open up about the event and the resulting feelings may help these to be processed.

BOX 37.5 Case Example

When Clarissa is four years old, her mother contacts her health visitor for advice, as Clarissa has started to wet and soil, having previously been dry and clean both day and night. There have been no previous concerns about Clarissa's health or development.

The health visitor takes a brief history, which reveals that the family has recently moved house. This has entailed Clarissa moving from one nursery school to another, and she has told her mother how much she misses her friends at the old nursery, who now live too far away for her to visit easily. Clarissa has also confided in her mother how worried she is about making new friends and starting at proper school in a few months' time.

The health visitor advises Clarissa's mother to visit her general practitioner for a medical check up: to exclude, for instance, constipation or urinary tract infection. She discusses with Clarissa's mother the potential impact on Clarissa of the house move, with all the changes that have resulted for her. She explains that the developmental regression could well be part of this. She advises Clarissa's mother to continue to give Clarissa lots of tender loving care and plenty of opportunity to talk about her worries; plus exploring ways of supporting Carissa's friendships.

The health visitor gets the general practitioner to inform her of the outcome of the medical assessment, which shows that Clarissa's urine is free of infection and she does not appear to be constipated. The health visitor contacts Clarissa's mother by telephone a couple of months after their original meeting. Clarissa's mother describes having lots of chats with Clarissa to help her cope with all the changes in her life. She has taken Clarissa on a visit to her best friend at the old nursery, and a return visit is planned. She has made a point of meeting with the other mothers at the new nursery, to explore opportunities for inviting new friends home, especially those who are due to move to the same school at the same time. The soiling and wetting have not yet stopped completely, but have become a great deal better.

BOX 37.6 Case Example

Vikesh is 15 years old when he visits the community school nurse at her drop-in clinic to say that he feels like taking an overdose because his girlfriend of a year, Martha, has just dumped him. The nurse takes a deep breath, tries not to show how worried she is that Vikesh may kill himself, and helps Vikesh explain the situation to her.

It emerges that Vikesh does not want his parents to know that he has been having sex with Martha, who is still only 14 years old (Vikesh's parents do not in any case approve of his having a white girlfriend). They have been using contraception, but one day the condom burst, and Martha became pregnant. Vikesh was very upset that Martha arranged for an abortion without asking him first. Since then, things have been difficult between them, with lots of arguments, and Martha has just announced that she cannot stand it any longer. Since then, Vikesh has found it difficult to get to sleep and wakes up frequently, with difficulty getting back to sleep. His concentration at school has plummeted: he used to get A's and B's, but is now getting C's and D's.

The community school nurse says she would like to refer him to CAMHS, as she is concerned he may be depressed and might harm himself, but Vikesh refuses, as he is convinced this will mean his parents finding out about everything. She mentions that he might get better more quickly if he takes some antidepressant tablets, but Vikesh says he definitely does not want any such thing, so she backtracks. She says she thinks it is important that Vikesh has someone to talk to regularly, particularly as he can't confide in his parents; and she isn't in a position to offer this herself but could ask the school counsellor to see Vikesh.

Vikesh is not keen on seeing someone new, but reluctantly agrees to seeing both of them together for an initial meeting, which fortunately the nurse is able to arrange for the next day. She negotiates with Vikesh what he will let her tell the school counsellor, and he says it will be all right to say about his splitting up with Martha, but he does not want her to tell him about the abortion. Vikesh also agrees that he will not take an overdose for the time being, since he can see that talking about things may help.

Fortunately, the introductory meeting goes well, and Vikesh agrees to see the school counsellor regularly, initially twice per week. It emerges that his parents have been having their own employment and marital difficulties. Vikesh still won't let them be informed about his distress. He gets steadily better over the next six months, despite not getting back together with Martha.

ASSESSMENT

As post-traumatic stress disorder is different in children compared to adults, developmental factors should be taken into account in its assessment, and treatment needs to be adapted according to the child's age and developmental stage.[15]

Sensitivity is required in relation to probing into traumatic events, particularly those that are private and secret, such as sexual abuse or domestic violence. Events with more public access, such as group catastrophes or road traffic accidents, are generally easier to talk about. In general, talking can help process the associated emotions, but sometimes it may raise the level of distress to unmanageable levels, in which case any pressure to reveal further details is likely to be counterproductive. This can then lead to difficulties with assessment and treatment, as it may not be at all clear what has actually happened, and what impact it may have had. The following two case examples are at either extreme of this continuum. In Box 37.7, Shazad finds even an intensive but very time-limited bit of talking about his trauma as part of his assessment helps him get better, and is more-or-less curative – unintentionally. In Box 37.8, professionals find Evelyn very difficult to help, because it seems impossible for her to speak about what has happened, and it is not even certain that significant trauma has occurred.

BOX 37.7 Case Example

A seven-year-old boy, Shazad, and his family are assessed by a child psychiatrist for a compensation claim two years after a road traffic accident. The child psychiatrist is unable to predict when the symptoms of post-traumatic stress disorder will resolve, so he arranges to see Shazad and his family one year later. Shazad's parents say that most of his symptoms have subsided, and, to the child psychiatrist's surprise, attribute this to the long discussion they had as part of the initial assessment. Shazad has not had any formal therapy, and his parents found the questions asked about the accident helped them to understand the impact it must have had on Shazad, and helped him to move on from it. In particular, the discussion in the first interview seemed to free up the family to talk about the accident – they no longer feared that talking about it would add to Shazad's difficulties.

BOX 37.8 Case Example

Evelyn presents at the age of nine years with restrictive anorexia nervosa that proves intractable over the next few years. Her drawings and the relationship she is observed to have with her father suggest to professionals that she has probably been sexually abused, or suffered some similar trauma. However, Evelyn never makes a disclosure, so no action can be taken. She does not respond well to therapy directed at her eating disorder, but survives with prolonged inpatient treatment. Advice from a specialist centre recommends that the impact of the trauma should somehow be addressed, but Evelyn never allows this to happen.

Begin by finding out who is concerned about what and what the family wants or expects from you. Then take a ***brief history*** of the precipitating event(s), gathering as much information as the child and family feel comfortable sharing at this stage. A simple question such as '*Tell me what happened*' can be a useful introduction. Ask ***who has been affected*** by the trauma and ***how***, as in many cases more than one family member is affected.

Find out if there are any ***legal proceedings*** pending and what the family's expectations may be about compensation or therapy: at times, the two can pull in opposite directions. Clarify whether you are being asked to do an assessment for court proceedings, in which case you will need a letter of instruction from a solicitor representing the child or an equivalent professional organisation. Clarify whether you are being asked for assessment as a prelude to treatment. Ideally, these two should not be done by the same person, but inevitably they may overlap (as in the case example in Box 37.7 above). One sort of conflict between the two arises because the worse the child's condition, the more compensation will be paid by the insurance company in the case of an accident, so there can at times (for some families or individuals) be a powerful motivator *not* to get better (this is sometimes labelled '***compensation neurosis***'). Another sort of conflict arises ***when a court case is pending***, for instance in a case of alleged sexual abuse or physical assault. Even assessment may prejudice the outcome of such a case if it includes discussion of the events that will be disputed in court – which it may be rather difficult to avoid if you want to do an adequate assessment and if you decide to provide treatment. This leads to a risk of preventing a successful prosecution because of the need for therapy, and in some cases of having the notes of your assessment or therapy sessions demanded (subpoenaed) by the court to establish what you have been talking about with the child and whether this could affect the evidence presented in court. It is hardly fair on the child to assure her of confidentiality when this revelation of everything to everyone in the courtroom is a possibility, but warning her of what the court may demand can make it very difficult for her to establish confidence in the therapeutic relationship.

In this sort of thorny area, it is as well to ask for as much advice from colleagues, managers, employers' solicitors and others as possible, and if appropriate to contact the Crown Prosecution Service for guidance prior to commencing therapy. It is sometimes possible to agree a compromise whereby you will continue to see the child for some support up until the court case, but will not discuss in your sessions any of the disputed evidence – until after the completion of the court hearing. This compromise can sometimes be satisfactory, as in the case example in Box 37.9, but often a victim may be so traumatised by her experiences that she has more difficulty than Helen in sticking to the boundaries agreed for the therapeutic sessions. An emotionally damaged victim may also find it difficult to give a coherent and convincing account of what has happened, and the evidence may seem insubstantial when challenged by a skilled defence barrister, so the prosecution fails, and the child feels very let down by the criminal justice system.

BOX 37.9 Case Example

Helen, aged 13, has alleged to social services and the police that she was raped on three occasions by her mother's cohabitee, Gavin, before he left the family home two months ago. There is medical evidence consistent with this, but Gavin denies all the allegations, saying that the worst that happened was that he walked into the bathroom by accident one day when Helen was fully undressed and in the bath. Helen's mother says she was aware there was tension between the two of them, but thought this was no more than the expected level of disagreement between a teenage girl and her 'stepfather'. She admits she left Helen and Gavin alone in the house more than she would have wished, because of her unsociable working hours. Because Helen's videotaped interview was very convincing to the police, the Crown Prosecution Service has decided to take the matter to court.

In the meantime, without discussing it with social services, Helen's general practitioner has referred her to the primary mental health worker for 'counselling', as she is understandably very distressed about the whole thing. The primary mental health worker does a preliminary assessment – without, however, going through any of the details that Helen has described in the videotape. She takes advice from her colleagues and line manager, discusses the situation with Helen's social worker, and comes back to Helen to say that she thinks Helen's situation is too complicated for her, and she needs to refer Helen to CAMHS. Once Helen has established what this means, she says she definitely does *not* want to be passed on!

Somewhat reluctantly, but with Helen's full agreement, the primary mental health worker contacts the Crown Prosecution Service, whose representative explains that the videotaped evidence is very important, but that it is likely the court will want Helen to be cross-examined by video link, as her account forms the bulk of the evidence. The medical evidence suggests that vaginal penetration was forced, but could be due to Helen having a sexual relationship with a peer, which she denies. The primary mental health worker agrees not to discuss with Helen anything that happened between her and Gavin prior to the court case, although she anticipates this may be difficult. She doesn't think it would be fair to deprive Helen of the opportunity for therapy altogether, and the representative of the Crown Prosecution Service agrees, so they arrange to meet weekly.

As it turns out, Helen is not at all keen on going through the details of what happened between her and Gavin with the primary mental health worker, as she feels she has unburdened herself of all this in front of the video camera and is aware that she will have to do the same in court. She is therefore content to be 'held' by talking about other areas of her life. She is hoping for a successful prosecution, as she feels that without this she might as well not have bothered to reveal to anyone what happened, and she is keen to have some sort of official acknowledgement of what she has been through.

Helen might have been disappointed, due to the strength of evidence required to convince a jury, but before the allotted court date, the daughter of a previous cohabitee of Gavin's, having heard through mutual friends what Helen has alleged, makes similar allegations. Although these are somewhat less convincing - due to being further in the past - the jury is impressed by some similarities in the two accounts of what Gavin is alleged to have done and by the prosecution being able to establish that the girls have neither met nor communicated in any way before meeting in court. When the postponed court case eventually takes place, the jury convicts Gavin by a majority of 10:2. Helen feels so much better after this that she requires only another three therapy sessions before she says she can manage on her own.

Cases without court involvement are generally easier to manage. The following components may contribute to an effective assessment.

➤ Consider seeing the ***young person alone***, without her parents. Some children may prefer to speak about inner experiences without parents present. This may be due to a number of possible reasons:
  — wanting to protect her parents
  — being fearful of her parents' reaction
  — feelings of intense shame or self-blame relating to the trauma
  — not feeling safe to express her feelings
  — being fearful of the strength or consequences of her own feelings
  — trying not to think about what happened, due to a desire to suppress painful memories.

➤ Other children may prefer to go through the details of the trauma with the comfort and security of familiar adults, who can also contribute important parts of the story, particularly if they have been present at the time of the precipitating event, for instance in the car when it crashed.

➤ Consider seeing the ***parent(s) alone***, without the young person. Parents too may be trying hard to avoid discussing the trauma, fearing this will distress their child and make things worse. Consider how the parents have been affected: they may be experiencing a strong emotional reaction, such as anger or guilt, in relation to what their child has experienced.

➤ It may be useful to meet with different ***family*** members separately either because several have been involved in the traumatic event; or because some have and some haven't; and because each has a different perspective. In a family in which multiple members have experienced the same or similar trauma (such as sexual abuse) it may be helpful to move on to seeing the whole family together (*see* Chapter 8 on Family Issues).

➤ *Allow sufficient time* for:
  — anyone who has traumatic experiences to recount to do so
  — each to explain how this makes her feel
  — each to regain her composure before ending the meeting with you.

➤ This will help each one feel heard, feel safe about sharing the information, and feel able to leave any difficult emotions behind. If this process is rushed, so that someone leaves in mid-flow or still distressed, it will be more difficult for her to engage in a similar process in the future, and she may spurn any further help or intervention that is offered.

➤ *Be aware of your own emotional responses.* Anyone who is unaffected emotionally by listening to a graphic account of a traumatic event is not truly listening. It is important however to remain calm and to be circumspect about expressing your own feelings. Although self-disclosure can sometimes be helpful in promoting engagement, the focus must remain on the client's emotional responses rather than the therapist's. Don't tell her you know how she feels: you don't. Don't try to minimise the experience, for instance by saying: 'Surely it isn't really that bad?' Don't comment on how *lucky* a family member may have been to escape significant harm. The converse is more likely to chime with the client's feelings: she was *unlucky* to experience the event in the first place; and many survivors feel extremely guilty about not having suffered as much as some others.

➤ You cannot expect the core features of post-traumatic stress disorder to emerge when you just listen. You should have a list of the diagnostic features by you (*see* Table 37.1 and the above definition of post-traumatic stress disorder in children) so that you can check whether or not the child has experienced each one by **asking specifically** about them. The young person may not have told anyone about some of these features for fear that:
— she is going mad
— she will relive the experience and it will feel worse
— others will not understand
— someone will tell her just to 'Pull yourself together'
— someone will say she should be glad to be alive
— she will exacerbate her survivor guilt.

➤ Sharing the contents of such a list with the client can be very reassuring for her: it shows that she is not alone in having such symptoms, which to some extent are to be expected. Far from going mad, she is merely experiencing what a proportion of individuals will experience after any similar trauma (about one in three after a severe event).

➤ The situation **prior to the trauma**, or previous similar events, may affect the child's response.
— Did the child have any recognised developmental or learning difficulties?
— Was the child resilient or sensitive?
— Has the child experienced a similar trauma before?
— Does anyone in the family have previous experience of a similar trauma?

➤ The **nature of the trauma** may affect the child's response:
— the intensity and duration of the event
— its suddenness or unexpectedness
— being trapped
— how many other people have been affected and to what extent.

➤ What happens **following the trauma** may affect the child's response.
— How are family and friends coping?
— Is there a supportive network around the child?
— Is there any continued threat of harm (such as aftershocks following an earthquake)?

MANAGEMENT AND REFERRAL

Research has shown that forcing everyone to have therapy after a traumatic event is unhelpful,[16] so single-session debriefing (discussion of all the horrible things that happened) should *not* be offered indiscriminately. If however symptoms are severe or persist for more than a month, then trauma-focused psychological treatment should be offered. In general, this should be individual and weekly (usually for 8-12 weeks), and so may require referral, particularly as sessions may need to last up to 90 minutes and involve cognitive techniques to help the young person adapt to the distressing memories. This can be very effective, however long ago the trauma occurred.

Eye movement desensitisation and reprocessing (**EMDR**) can also be very effective and may lead to a more rapid recovery. EMDR is a technique that uses bilateral stimulation such as encouraging an affected person to move their eyes from left to right across their visual field whilst concentrating intensely on the most upsetting parts of the traumatic memory (so is not suitable for young people who are not yet ready to think about what happened). How this helps is still unclear, but it has been explained using a model of the way the brain processes information.[17] If distressing experiences are not adequately processed, they remain in an undigested form that causes symptoms such as flashbacks, avoidance or increased arousal – which continue until some way can be found to work through them. EMDR may somehow facilitate the necessary work of making emotional sense of the traumatic experience, so accelerating information processing and allowing adaptive resolution of the traumatic memories. It may sound like a bizarre way to bypass conscious reflection, but it has been shown to work.[18]

There is sometimes a *dilemma* about the provision of therapy for post-traumatic stress disorder and its lesser variants, which is related to the spectrum of responses (*see* Figure 37.1). Milder symptoms improve best without any professional intervention. Moderate symptoms may improve best if the child has the opportunity to talk about her experiences –ideally with someone who can be sufficiently unaffected to be able to listen actively (this does not *have* to be a professional: *see* case example in Box 37.10). Severe symptoms may be very painful or difficult to talk about, so that the child may not wish to engage in any form of talking therapy. This may be related to the child's cognitive capacity and verbal abilities, or simply to the subjective severity of the trauma. For some of these children, eye movement desensitisation and reprocessing may be more acceptable, if it is available locally.[19] For others, several sessions of individual therapy may be needed to build up trust before any attempt is made to talk about what happened (so there may need to be more than 12 sessions).

For yet others, the time may not be right to embark on therapy, and it may simply have to wait until the young person is ready. The dilemma here is that therapeutic talking (or eye movement desensitisation and reprocessing) enables some *processing* of the events and associated emotions, so that they no longer have such power to cause distress and impairment (for instance through nightmares, flashbacks, dissociation . . .). By *not* processing the experiences, the child is allowing them to have continued power, for instance through *avoidance* of anything that reminds her of what happened, which can in turn result in the development of new fears or anxieties.

There are **indirect ways** of trying to resolve this dilemma: activities such as semi-structured art activities, storytelling, pictures and puppetry can all be used as aids to recall, especially with preschool and latency children.[20] An older child or adolescent may find it helpful to express herself in some creative way, such as painting, drawing, singing, making music, taking part in drama or writing (prose, poetry or songs). Unfortunately, these may not on their own be enough to achieve adequate resolution, and such activities are probably best used to **facilitate** rather than replace the therapeutic process.[21] In practical terms, this means that referral may still be necessary.

BOX 37.10 Case Example

Samuel, aged eight years old, and his mother become the victims of an assault and robbery while on holiday in France. Samuel witnesses his mother being held around the throat and threatened with a knife until she hands over all the money and jewellery that she has on her. Samuel is meanwhile restrained by another attacker and told that he will be hurt unless his mother complies.

On their return to the UK, Samuel's mother visits her general practitioner to ask for some help for both of them. She says she is having fewer difficulties than Samuel but is struggling to help him talk about what happened: every time she tries, he says he is not really bothered and won't talk. The general practitioner encourages Samuel's mother to help him talk about the attack in whatever way she can and also asks the primary mental health worker to meet with them both.

When the primary mental health worker meets with Samuel and his mother a month later, she reports that Samuel has already significantly improved. Samuel has been able to speak regularly to his maternal grandfather, with whom he has always been very close. When they meet alone as part of the assessment, Samuel tells the primary mental health worker that he was reluctant to speak to his mother about the assault, as he was worried it would upset her too much. He has noticed his mother crying when she thinks she is alone, and not going out as much as before the attack. She subsequently reveals to the primary mental health worker that she feels very isolated and fearful for her safety.

From the assessment, it is apparent that Samuel's mother is experiencing post-traumatic stress disorder: unlike Samuel's, her symptoms are not subsiding. Given Samuel's progress, the primary mental health worker says she will not make another appointment to see Samuel, but will do so within the next six months if necessary. She obtains his mother's agreement to refer her to adult mental health services for cognitive behavioural therapy.

Other interventions may also aid recovery.
➤ Explaining to family members what may happen following a traumatic event (**psychoeducation**). Children often show symptoms such as increased anxiety, worsening behaviour and regression that in general will get better in

time – providing the distressing events do not continue. Parents should be encouraged to give additional tender loving care until the emotional disturbance has subsided, but not to relax limits on behaviour. Parental *guilt* about what the child has been through (however irrational) may make it difficult to be firm and consistent, but this is what children need, in addition to support and understanding. Another pitfall for parents is to underestimate the emotional impact on the child of life events that adults may be able to take in stride, such as a house move or the departure of a friend. A child mental health professional may be able to help parents see the situation from the child's perspective.

➤ *Practical advice* may help some families. Examples include:
— suggestions on how to ameliorate the effects of parental separation (*see* Chapter 9)
— how to be effective in helping prevent the continuation of bullying (*see* Chapter 22)
— ensuring that all family members who require treatment have access to it (*see* case example in Box 37.10)
— providing sources of written information (*see* 'Resources' below)
— providing information about local support groups.

➤ It may be helpful to *involve parents and other family members in therapy* – despite the lack of hard evidence for this.[22] How best to do this depends on the individual circumstances.
— Parents may be able to help children by *facilitating discussions* of what happened. This may however be difficult for parents who have suffered in the same event (such as a family car crash), or a similar experience (such as childhood sexual abuse), or in cases where the trauma has been so severe that any account would be difficult to listen to. It may be easier in milder situations, such as an acute stress reaction or adjustment disorder.
— Help the child deal with *avoidance, anxiety or fears*. Anxiety management strategies may be useful (*see* Chapter 20). Once parents understand the way symptoms may be maintained by avoidance (or even increased if new fears develop), they are more likely to make sense of the child's behaviour, help her to stop avoiding situations, and prevent further fears from developing.

➤ *Referral to social services* may be necessary if any of the following apply:
— sexual abuse may have been perpetrated by a family member
— carers seem unable to protect the child from further abuse
— there is evidence of domestic violence
— the home environment is chaotic, neglectful or in other ways unsafe.

➤ *Referral to specialist CAMHS* may be necessary if any of the following apply:
— the young person has significant depressive symptoms
— the young person is at risk of serious self-harm
— the young person appears to be using drugs and/or alcohol as a coping mechanism
— the trauma involved serious injury or death to a significant loved one
— the child's carers appear are too distressed themselves to offer adequate support to the child.

➤ A different approach may be needed for ***disasters*** affecting large numbers of people. This should be adequately described in a local disaster management plan,[23] which should specify how health, social services and education may each have complementary roles in organising appropriate social and psychological support for those affected by a disaster. For instance, when the community affected is an individual school (*see* case example in Box 37.11), support and debriefing services can be provided by professionals already known to the school such as educational psychologists and primary mental health workers. A disaster plan should have the following components:
— immediate practical help
— support for the affected community in caring for all those involved in the disaster
— assessment of everyone involved in the disaster after one month in order to identify those who *would* benefit from therapy, since the immediate provision of single-session debriefing is not recommended.

➤ ***Refugees or asylum-seekers*** and their children arriving in the UK are likely to have experienced major trauma, so may also benefit from a screening programme. The need for interpreters may complicate the assessment. The efficacy of treatment may be improved if bicultural therapists are available, but in any case every effort should be made to understand the foreign culture and the circumstances giving rise to the trauma.[24]

BOX 37.11 Case Example

An arson attack on a primary school during a half-term holiday has destroyed the classrooms used for Year 3 and 4: the classes will have to relocate temporarily to the local secondary school while repairs take place. Pet gerbils have died in the fire. Much of the work done in preparation for the school's annual play has been ruined.

The head teacher is concerned about what to tell her pupils and in what way: she is aware that the fire has been on the local news and that many rumours have spread through the community. She therefore meets with the school's educational psychologist and community school nurse before the end of the half-term break to discuss how to inform the pupils. They decide that the head teacher will speak to the whole school in assembly on the first day back after half-term. The educational psychologist advises that it will probably be important to give the children an age-appropriate description of the fire and the preliminary plans for repairs. He suggests that it may be best to enable informal discussion of the fire amongst peers by providing the known facts and allowing a few questions during the assembly but probably not to allow the assembly to turn into a mass debriefing session.

The head teacher decides to explain to the assembled pupils that it would be understandable for some of them to feel quite emotional about what has happened: they may for instance feel shock, sadness, fear or anger. She will reassure everyone that such emotions are to be expected when something so awful has happened. The community school nurse suggests that she and the teacher with responsibility for pastoral care should make themselves available during the lunch-break for the next two weeks, in case any pupils want to drop in to discuss the impact of the fire. A newsletter containing all the same information will be distributed to all parents so that they are aware of what their children know.

BOX 37.12 Practice Points for dealing with trauma

During an assessment, gather as much information about the precipitating traumatic event as the child (or parent) is able to share.

During an assessment, offer to see the child separately, and give the same opportunity to parents.

When discussing stressful or traumatic events, allow sufficient time for the child to compose herself before she leaves the session.

Be aware that more than one family member may be affected and may need support, or referral.

Encourage processing of the events – but only to the extent that this is tolerable. Refer for therapy if you feel unable to provide this yourself.

RESOURCES

Websites

- The Royal College of Psychiatrists has two leaflets on post-traumatic stress disorder, one brief and one longer; and one on how to cope after a trauma: www.rcpsych.ac.uk/mentalhealthinfo/problems/ptsd/ptsdkeyfacts.aspx
- www.rcpsych.ac.uk/mentalhealthinfo/problems/ptsd/posttraumaticstressdisorder.aspx
- www.rcpsych.ac.uk/mentalhealthinfo/problems/ptsd/copingafteratraumaticevent.aspx
- The charity Young Minds also has an information leaflet about post-traumatic stress disorder on its website: www.youngminds.org.uk/my-head-hurts/treatments/mental-health-difficulties/post-traumatic-stress-disorder-ptsd
- ASSIST – Assistance Support & Self-help in Surviving Trauma – is a UK-based support and information resource for people suffering from post-traumatic stress disorder: www.assisttraumacare.org.uk

Books for children and families

- Herbert C, Wetmore A. *Overcoming Traumatic Stress*. New York: Basic Books; 2008.
- Kennerley H. *Overcoming Childhood Trauma*. London: Robinson Publishing; 2000.
- Lewis D. *Helping Your Anxious Child*. UK: Vermilion; 2002.
- Lovett J. *Small Wonders: healing childhood trauma with EMDR*. New York, NY: The Free Press; 1999.
  For parents and professionals, this book illustrates how EMDR can be used with trauma and a wide range of other difficulties.

Books for professionals

- Smith P, Perrin S, Yule W, *et al. Post Traumatic Stress Disorder (CBT with Children, Adolescents and Families)*. London: Routledge; 2009.
- Tinker RH, Wilson S. *Through the Eyes of a Child: EMDR with children*. New York, NY: Norton Professional Books; 1999.
  This book demystifies the use of EMDR with children, and has lots of case examples with trauma and other problems.

REFERENCES

1 Scheeringa MS, Zeanah CH, Drell MJ, *et al.* Two approaches to the diagnosis of post-traumatic stress disorder in infancy and early childhood. *J Am Acad Child Adolesc Psychiatry.* 1995; **34**(2): 191–200.

2 Yule W. Posttraumatic stress disorder in children and adolescents. *International Review of Psychiatry.* 2001; **13**: 194–200.

3 Bauer PJ, Kroupina MG, Schwade JA, *et al.* If memory serves, will language? Later verbal accessibility of early memories. *Dev Psychopathol.* 1998; **10**(4): 655–79.

4 Cohen JA. Practice parameters for the assessment and treatment of children and adolescents with post-traumatic stress disorder. *J Am Acad Child Adolesc Psychiatry.* 1998; **37**(10): 4–26.

5 Piaget J. Piaget's theory. In: Mussen PH, editor. *Carmichael's Manual of Child Psychology (Volume 1).* New York, NY: Wiley; 1970. pp. 703–32.

6 Goodyer IM, Herbert J, Tamplin A, *et al.* Recent life events, cortisol, dehydroepiandrosterone and the onset of major depression in high-risk adolescents. *Br J Psychiatry.* 2000; **177**: 499–504.

7 Perrin S, Smith P, Yule W. The assessment and treatment of post-traumatic stress disorder in children and adolescents. *J Child Psychol Psychiatry.* 2000; **41**(3): 277–89.

8 Terr LC. Chowchilla revisited: The effects of psychic trauma of four years after a schoolbus kidnapping. *Am J Psychiatry.* 1983; **140**(12): 1543–50.

9 Dollinger SJ, O'Donnell JP, Staley AA. Lightning-strike disaster: effects on children's fears and worries. *J Consult Clin Psychol.* 1984; **52**(6): 1028–38.

10 Terr LC. Childhood traumas: an outline and overview. *Am J Psychiatry.* 1991; **148**(1): 10–20.

11 Cohen, op. cit.

12 Yule W. Post-traumatic stress disorder in child survivors of shipping disasters: the sinking of the *Jupiter. Psychotherapy and Psychosomatics.* 1992; **57**: 200–5.

13 Mirza KA, Bhadrinath BR, Goodyer IM, *et al.* Post-traumatic stress disorder in children and adolescents following road traffic accidents. *Br J Psychiatry.* 1998; **172**: 443–7.

14 Pynoos RS, Goenjian A, Tashjian M, *et al.* Post-traumatic stress reactions in children after the 1988 Armenian earthquake. *Br J Psychiatry.* 1993; **163**: 239–47.

15 Salmon K, Bryant RA. Post-traumatic stress disorder in children: the influence of developmental factors. *Clinical Psychology Review.* 2002; **22**: 163–88.

16 National Collaborating Centre for Mental Health. *Post-traumatic stress disorder (PTSD): the management of PTSD in adults and children in primary and secondary care* [Clinical Guideline number 26]. London: National Institute for Health and Clinical Excellence; 2005. Available at: http://guidance.nice.org.uk/CG26/NiceGuidance/pdf (accessed 4 April 2011).

17 Shapiro F, Maxfield L. Eye Movement Desensitization and Reprocessing (EMDR): information processing in the treatment of trauma. *Journal of Clinical Psychology.* 2002; **58**(8): 933–46.

18 Adler-Tapia R, Settle C. Evidence of the efficacy of EMDR with children and adolescents in individual psychotherapy: a review of the research published in peer-reviewed journals. *Journal of EMDR Practice and Research.* 2009; **3**(4): 232–47.

19 www.emdrassociation.org.uk/findatherapist.htm

20 Salmon, op. cit.

21 Bunjevac T, Kuterovac G. Report on the results of psychological evaluation of the art therapy program in schools in Hercegovina. Zagreb: UNICEF; 1994.

22 National Collaborating Centre for Mental Health, op. cit.

23 Ibid.

24 Ibid.

CHAPTER 38

Traumatic brain injury

INTRODUCTION

Head injury due to trauma (most commonly a road traffic accident) can cause difficulties in three ways: it could be said to be a form of *triple jeopardy*.

► The child's *pre-existing conditions* will continue to cause problems, amplified by the effects of the head injury. For instance, any specific learning difficulty is likely to be more difficult to cope with. The core symptoms of ADHD, particularly impulsivity and hyperactivity, make children accident prone, as anyone working in Accident and Emergency can confirm. Such children are more likely to bang their heads or be knocked over by an unseen car, so they have a higher than average risk of head injury.[1,2] Any pre-existing ADHD is likely to be more severe after a significant head injury (it may have been undiagnosed before).

► The acute and chronic effects of the injury have an impact similar to *any chronic illness or disability* (*see* Chapter 42 on Chronic Paediatric Illness).

► Added to both of these are the specific consequences of the injury that result from it being *to the brain*. These may include, for instance:
  — overall cognitive deficit
  — visuo-spatial difficulties (particularly parietal lobe damage)
  — memory difficulties (particularly in temporal lobe damage)
  — disinhibition (particularly in frontal lobe damage)
  — personality change
  — behavioural difficulties (but these are likely to be due to a combination of all three factors).

BOX 38.1 Case Example

Anthony is seven years old when he is knocked down by a car while crossing the road. Scans show widespread bruising to the brain, and also a blood clot on the right side of his brain that is gradually enlarging, and has to be surgically removed. He remains unconscious for three days and on the paediatric intensive care unit for a week.

Subsequent paediatric assessment reveals that he has a left-sided weakness which completely resolves over the next six months. He develops epilepsy, which proves difficult to control with anticonvulsants. He is thought to have ADHD, but a trial of medication is delayed pending adequate control of his fits. At school, his behavioural problems are a great deal worse than before the accident, and he struggles to make academic progress. His mother also struggles to manage him and his two siblings at home as well as running a corner shop with her partner. Eventually, a full assessment of educational needs enables him to be transferred to a special school for behavioural, emotional and social problems, where he is much happier.

BOX 38.2 Case Example

Robert is five years old when he falls out of a second-floor window while playing with his elder sister, who has recently been diagnosed with ADHD. He spends 17 days on a ventilator, during which his separated parents are told that he nearly died. He has a very prolonged recovery. Five years later, he is managing adequately at a special school for moderate learning difficulties. He also benefits from medication for ADHD in the form of methylphenidate.

Many cases will be less severe than in the two case examples in Boxes 38.1 and 38.2; this chapter focuses on the mildest form of head injury, as this seems to give rise to most confusion for families and professionals.

Concussion

This can be loosely defined as bruising of the brain without large-scale structural damage, and the term may be used in a non-professional sense to refer to a brief loss of consciousness. It is the mildest form of head injury and can also be known as mild traumatic brain injury. Loss of consciousness may or may not occur. More severe head injury is likely to be accompanied by longer periods of unconsciousness or coma (defined inclusively as *a sleep-like state in which a person is not conscious*).[3] Another more formal definition of concussion is:

> The common result of a blow to the head or sudden deceleration usually causing an altered mental state, either temporary or prolonged. Physiological and/or anatomical disruption of connections between some nerve cells in the brain may occur.[4]

The symptoms are *usually* transient, lasting only days or weeks, and can be divided into biological, cognitive and affective (emotional).
Biological symptoms
➤ Headache
➤ Dizziness
➤ Nausea or vomiting
➤ Poor motor coordination

➤ Difficulty balancing
➤ Lethargy
➤ Changes in sleep patterns
➤ Restlessness
➤ Light sensitivity
➤ Seeing bright lights
➤ Blurred vision
➤ Double vision
➤ Tinnitus (ringing in the ears).

Cognitive symptoms
➤ Difficulty concentrating
➤ Confusion or disorientation
➤ Difficulty with reasoning
➤ Difficulty performing everyday activities
➤ Post-traumatic amnesia: forgetting what happened for a period *after* the head injury
➤ Pre-traumatic amnesia: forgetting what happened for a period *before* the head injury
➤ Difficulty with everyday activities.

Affective symptoms
➤ Loss of interest in favorite activities or items
➤ Irritability or crankiness
➤ Tearfulness
➤ Displays of emotion that are inappropriate or out of proportion.

Most cases of concussion resolve completely without any long-lasting effects. However, a few seem to leave some persisting loss of function or change in personality, possibly because of undetected persisting subtle brain damage – this can be called '*post-concussional syndrome*'. Long-term symptoms may include headache, dizziness, memory deficits, slowness of thought, poor concentration, communication problems, inability to work and problems with self-care.[5]

In these cases, the young person and his family may have some difficulty understanding and accepting these changes, particularly the altered personality. The family and particularly the parents may need help in adjusting their expectations for the child's future life. The loss of the expected child and the substitution of a different child may sometimes lead to strong grief reactions.

A case example in which it seems possible that some symptoms might have persisted is described in Box 38.3.

Boxing

Boxing can cause various injuries (*see* Box 38.4),[6] which have led the British Medical Association to campaign for it to be banned, starting with a ban for children under 16 years, who are most likely to be unaware of the risks such as long-term brain

BOX 38.3 Case Example

Manilka, aged 13 years, is referred to the primary mental health worker by her general practitioner because of deteriorating behaviour at home and at school. She is getting into conflict with her (non-identical) twin sister, her younger brother and their parents, and swearing at her teachers. The primary mental health worker takes a family and developmental history. She is struck by how different Manilka seems to be from her twin sister, so asks when their parents first noticed such a difference. At first the parents say it was when the twins both started entering puberty, about two years ago. Then they remember that Manilka was knocked down by a car while crossing the road on the way back from school, which was also about two years ago. She was taken to Accident and Emergency, by which time she had recovered consciousness; she was kept in overnight for observation, but had no broken bones. She seemed a bit different for a week or two afterwards, and had a bit of a headache and some dizziness for a couple of days, but no vomiting or other symptoms. She eventually remembered the point at which she had begun to cross the road, but could never remember anything between the head injury and her arrival in hospital, although the ambulance drivers said that she regained consciousness within the ambulance.

As Manilka's parents discuss this with the primary mental health worker, they begin to remember that Manilka began to clash with other people soon after this head injury, and seemed more disinhibited: more likely to do things without thinking of the effect on other people and say things that normally she would have kept to herself.

Paediatric assessment as to whether there are any long-lasting sequelae to the head injury is inconclusive. The primary mental health worker cannot be sure that the head injury is the main reason for Manilka's current behaviour, but it seems a potential explanation for at least some of it.

impairment and may therefore be unable to give informed consent. The argument is that there is no place in contemporary society for a youth sport whose primary goal is to give your opponent concussion. In addition, there is evidence to contradict the commonly held view that violent sports channel young people's aggression in a prosocial way: on the contrary, power sports (boxing, wrestling and weight-lifting) actually seem to enhance antisocial behaviour (both violent and non-violent), possibly due to the 'macho' attitudes these sports encourage.[7] In contrast, oriental martial arts such as karate and judo, if pursued without the other power sports, do not seem to be associated with the same increase in antisocial behaviour, as would be expected from the non-violent philosophy often accompanying their tuition.

BOX 38.4 Injuries caused by boxing

Brain damage: the blows received during boxing cause the brain to move within the skull, damaging blood vessels, nerves and brain tissue. Even wearing a helmet does not necessarily prevent this.

Acute bleeding into the brain: this is the leading cause of boxing deaths.
Damage to eyes, ears and nose: boxing can sometimes cause loss of vision or hearing.

ASSESSMENT

If you find there is a history of head injury, it is worth finding out more about this before dismissing it as a self-limiting problem that has no effects lasting longer than a few weeks.

➤ What happened to cause the blow to the head?
➤ Was there a period of unconsciousness and if so, how long? The length of unconsciousness can be an index of severity.
➤ How long was the period of amnesia, before and/or after the accident? How much is forgotten can also be an index of severity.
➤ Were there any of the symptoms commonly seen in concussion?
➤ Were any brain scans done? If so, what did they show?
➤ Was any part of the brain more damaged than the rest?
➤ What changes in the child did close friends and family members notice immediately after the accident?
➤ What changes do they still notice?
➤ What impact have these changes had:
  — on the child?
  — on other family members?
  — on friends?
➤ What is the emotional reaction of the child and family when discussing the events that led to the head injury?
➤ Is there any evidence of post-traumatic stress disorder such as nightmares, flashbacks or avoidance of reminders? (*See* Chapter 37 on Adjustment Disorder and Post-Traumatic Stress Disorder.)

It is difficult (or perhaps impossible) to predict the likelihood of post-concussional syndrome on the basis of characteristics of the initial injury or its severity.[8]

MANAGEMENT AND REFERRAL

Often it may be enough to explain the child's behavioural and personality changes in terms of the head injury. Parents are often surprised at how long these changes can continue after the accident. A paediatric assessment should be arranged if this has not already been done. In some cases, specific management strategies may be required to address the problems presented, such as:

➤ psychometric testing (with a view to targeting extra help in school)
➤ behaviour management
➤ family therapy
➤ therapy for post-traumatic stress disorder or post traumatic symptoms (*see* Chapter 37)

➤ medication, for instance for epilepsy, ADHD symptoms or unmanageable aggressive outbursts.

Any of these may require referral.

Parents may benefit from ongoing support from professionals, supplemented if possible by national and/or local support services. Special educational provision may be required. If the child's difficulties are severe and affecting family function, periods of respite care for the child can give parents a much-needed break, and support the child's continued placement at home.

RESOURCES
Websites
- The Children's Brain Injury Trust: www.cbituk.org
- The Headway Brain Injury Association: www.headway.org.uk
- Information sheets from Great Ormond Street Children's Hospital: www.ich.ucl.ac.uk/gosh_families/information_sheets/head_injury/head_injury_families.html

Book for parents
- Powell T. *Head Injury: a practical guide.* 2nd ed. Milton Keynes: Speechmark Publishing; 2004.
  Although not specifically about children, this guide to the general principles of looking after head-injured people is packed with useful information and easy to read.

REFERENCES
1 Keenan HT, Hall GC, Marshall SW. Early head injury and attention-deficit/hyperactivity disorder: retrospective cohort study. *BMJ.* 2008; **337**: a1984.
2 Zwi M, Clamp P. Injury and attention-deficit/hyperactivity disorder: monitoring children with early injuries could reduce later risk. *BMJ.* 2008; **337**: a2244.
3 National Institute for Health and Clinical Excellence. Head Injury: *triage, assessment, investigation and early management of head injury in infants, children and adults* [Clinical Guideline number 56]. London: National Collaborating Centre for Acute Care; 2007. Available at: www.nice.org.uk/nicemedia/pdf/CG56guidance.pdf (accessed 5 April 2011).
4 National Institute for Health and Clinical Excellence, op. cit.
5 Ibid.
6 www.bma.org.uk/health_promotion_ethics/sports_exercise/boxing.jsp
7 Endresen IM, Olweus D. Participation in power sports and antisocial involvement in preadolescent and adolescent boys. *J Child Psychol Psychiatry.* 2005; **46**(5): 468–78.
8 National Institute for Health and Clinical Excellence, op. cit.

CHAPTER 39

Obsessive-compulsive disorder

INTRODUCTION

Obsessive-compulsive disorder (OCD) can affect children, adolescents and adults. It usually begins in childhood, can have serious developmental consequences, and can also cause significant distress. Obsessions and compulsions, rituals and habits are also part of normal childhood development. Many preschool children develop obsessive interests or have their own rituals – this is nothing to be alarmed about. A toddler or young child's interests in tractors, trains or cars can appear almost obsessional at times. However, as the child grows older, these interests usually pass or decrease and are replaced by other, more age-appropriate ones.

Like many of the other child mental health difficulties dealt with in this book, obsessions and compulsions need to be viewed on a continuum: ranging from age-appropriate obsessional behaviour and adherence to routines to severe intrusive, obsessional thoughts and associated compulsive behaviour that impair functioning, and so constitute a disorder.

One way of thinking about routines, rituals or habits is whether they are functional or non-functional. A *functional* routine is one that is useful and helps achieve a goal: for example, having a bedtime routine helps a child settle at night and a morning routine helps all members of the family get out of the house on time. *Non-functional* routines are time-consuming and usually achieve little in the external world – although they may have important rewards in the child's internal world (see below).

When are obsessions and compulsions abnormal?

These symptoms are said to be abnormal and constitute a disorder if they are:
➤ unwanted and causing distress
➤ time-consuming: taking up more than one hour a day
➤ interfering with functioning – for example, the child has difficulty getting out of the house on time each morning, or cannot go to social occasions.

Sometimes, such symptoms may be a consequence of another disorder, such as autistic spectrum disorder or depression: obsessive-compulsive disorder may not be the primary problem.

In adults, it may be easier to reach a diagnosis and come to a shared perception of these symptoms as a problem: firstly, an adult is usually more able to describe his symptoms; secondly, a child is less likely to have the kind of awareness that involves seeing his obsessions or compulsions as excessive or unreasonable.

Terminology

A number of different terms are used to describe the main features of obsessive-compulsive disorder. These are summarised in Table 39.1 below. An *obsession* is an unwanted, intrusive thought, image or urge that repeatedly enters the young

TABLE 39.1 The main features of obsessive-compulsive disorder

An **obsession** is a thought, idea, image or doubt with the following qualities:
  It is intrusive – it just pops into a young person's mind, interrupting his thoughts.
  It may be fleeting or persistent.
  It is usually unpleasant and unwanted.
  It usually prompts attempts to suppress, neutralise or ignore it – often unsuccessful.
  It is repeated – often many times.
  It can have characteristic themes, such as contamination, harm to others, sexual
    fantasies, impending disasters, counting or symmetry.
  It is often accompanied by a fear that something bad will happen.
  It can often lead to anxiety, guilt or shame. These in turn can prompt a compulsion.

A **compulsion** is a repetitive, purposeful behaviour or mental act with the following characteristics:
  There is a strong feeling or urge to carry out the compulsion.
  It often has to be carried out according to certain rules or in a set way.
  It may be very time-consuming.
  It may be accompanied by a fear that something awful will happen if the behaviour is
    not carried out.
  It can either be *overt* and so observable by others, such as washing, checking,
    touching, hoarding, ordering, arranging or asking questions; or a *covert* mental act
    that is hidden from others, such as counting or repeating a certain phrase silently:
    this can be called a *cognitive* compulsion.

Neutralising has the aim of undoing a perceived harm: for instance, it could consist
    of briefly forming a positive image to counter an intrusive negative image and so
    reduce the associated anxiety.
  It may have overt as well as covert elements, such as actions that reverse damage:
    for instance, rubbing a hand on one's trousers to undo the harm done by shaking
    someone else's hand.

A **ritual** can be synonymous with a compulsion, but it is usually a sequence of actions
    rather than a single action.

A **rumination** is a cyclical sequence of thoughts. It can be synonymous with an
    obsession or with brooding.
  It goes round and round without leading to any new insights.
  It can occur not only in obsessive-compulsive disorder, but also in depression, eating
    disorders and psychosis.

Avoidance is often associated with obsessive-compulsive disorder, although it is not
    part of the definition.
  Young people may avoid certain other people, places, objects or behaviours for fear of
    dangerous consequences, raising anxiety or triggering obsessions.
  For example, a young person with obsessions about germs and cleaning compulsions
    will usually strive to avoid any object or situation that he perceives as contaminating.

person's mind. *Compulsions* are repetitive behaviours or mental acts that the young person feels driven to perform.[1]

Obsessions and compulsions occur together in about 60% of individuals with a diagnosis of obsessive-compulsive disorder and may be fuelled by anxiety, guilt or shame.[2] This distress leads to a compulsive urge. If the compulsion is carried out, this reduces the distress. The reduction in distress is illustrated diagrammatically in Figure 39.1: it reinforces the repeated cycle of obsessions leading to compulsions. This does not apply to everyone: 40% of individuals can experience either obsessions or compulsions alone.

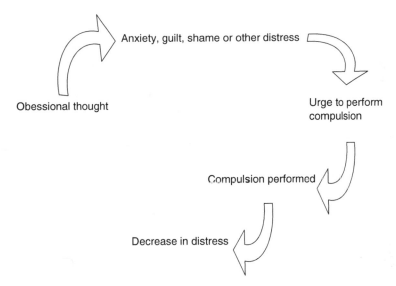

Anxiety, guilt, shame or other distress

Obessional thought

Urge to perform compulsion

Compulsion performed

Decrease in distress

FIGURE 39.1 The relation between obsessions, compulsions and the associated distress – how compulsive behaviours reduce distress, thus reinforcing and maintaining the problem

Prevalence

Obsessive-compulsive disorder is thought to occur in as much as 1–2% of the population,[3] but many may keep potentially embarrassing symptoms hidden from friends and family – so epidemiological figures may be underestimates. A young person is likely not to tell others about his obsessions or compulsions for fear of being thought 'bad' or 'mad'.

Intriguingly, the content of obsessional thoughts is often the very opposite of an individual's beliefs or moral values, so the resulting conflict can create a great deal of distress. For example, a religious young person may have unspeakable thoughts about God that he is sure are blasphemous; an adolescent who is firmly against war and violence may have thoughts of hurting or killing others; or a young person with no sexual experience who does not believe in sex before commitment may have bizarre sexual fantasies.

BOX 39.1 Case Example

Holly is referred at the age of 13 years to the primary mental health worker because of strange behaviour at school. The school has got to know Holly as a popular and sociable child since she joined the school at 11 years, but over the last six months she has become more socially isolated. At home, she has been using the bathroom with increasing frequency.

Holly admits to the primary mental health worker that she has been having horrible thoughts about other people pop into her mind repeatedly: she will not divulge the content of these thoughts, but does let slip the adjective 'disgusting'. She has found only two ways to make them go away: either to perform counting rituals such as counting in multiples of two or 80, or to use the toilet, even when she does not need to. She has started to think she must be a horrible person to have such thoughts, which constantly interfere with her concentration in class and during homework. She has not dared tell anyone about them, for fear someone will think her mad. Together with her diminishing self-esteem, this has contributed to her social isolation.

Who develops obsessive-compulsive disorder?

Whilst anyone may develop obsessive-compulsive disorder, it often runs in families and seems to have a strong genetic component. Obsessions and compulsions can also occur in a number of other conditions, for example:

➤ autistic spectrum disorder
➤ Tourette's syndrome
➤ anorexia nervosa
➤ depression
➤ psychosis.

Rarely but importantly, certain medical conditions seem to lead to obsessive-compulsive disorder, including the following:

➤ an auto-immune response to a streptococcal infection (most commonly a sore throat) that has been labelled paediatric autoimmune neuropsychiatric disorder associated with streptococcus (PANDAS)
➤ epilepsy
➤ systemic lupus erythematosis (SLE)
➤ traumatic brain injury
➤ brain tumours
➤ rheumatic fever.

In most cases, no apparent trigger, illness or cause can be found other than a familial vulnerability to anxiety, which may be genetic.

Obsessive-compulsive disorder presents more commonly in the early 20s than the under-18s, but 30–50% of adults recall a childhood onset.[4] Of children with obsessive-compulsive symptoms, 50–70% continue to have these as adults.[5] Obsessive-compulsive disorder can have a significant impact on a child's social functioning and academic performance at a time when he is developing and mastering new skills in these areas, which can result in long-term social and academic difficulties. These may include for instance school refusal, social anxiety or overall underachievement. Earlier recognition and treatment of obsessive-compulsive disorder, when symptoms have recently begun and are amenable to challenge, may reduce such negative sequelae and alleviate years of impairment.

ASSESSMENT

As mentioned above, a child may find it more difficult than an adult to describe his obsessions or compulsive thoughts, and may not have told anyone about them. Consequently it may be mainly the parents who present for help with inexplicable behaviour and the child may not perceive this as a problem.

Begin by finding out *who is worried about what* and whether the child has any other medical or developmental problems. If possible, spend some time talking to the child on his own, partly to ask what he has been thinking and doing. Aim to get as clear a description as possible of the nature and content of recurrent thoughts and the associated behaviours and feelings. Some examples of exploratory questions are given in Box 39.2.

BOX 39.2 Useful questions to ask in an assessment for obsessive-compulsive disorder

Are there any thoughts that keep bothering you that you just can't seem to get out of your mind?

Does your mind frequently make you count things, touch things or move things, even though you know you do not have to?

Do you find yourself checking things?

Do you find it difficult to cope with making mistakes?

Do you worry about saying or doing bad things, even though you don't actually do them?

Do you like to have things in a certain order, symmetrical or 'just right'?

Are you worried about contamination, for instance from dirt, animals, certain places or other people?

Do you have to wash yourself repeatedly?

Do you have to clean or tidy your bedroom repeatedly?

Do you have to clean or rearrange your possessions repeatedly?

Do you collect things or struggle to throw things away?

It may also be useful to ask these sorts of questions in the form of a brief rating scale such as the Short Obsessive-Compulsive Screener (*see* Table 39.2).[6] This can help the child describe what is going on and how much it is affecting him. It can also function (in non-specialist settings) as a screen for referral: a score of 6 or

TABLE 39.2 The Short Obsessive-Compulsive Screener (SOCS)

PLEASE ANSWER EACH QUESTION BY TICKING THE BOX THAT MOST APPLIES:			
Does your mind often make you do things – such as checking or touching things or counting things – even though you know you don't really have to?	No ☐	A bit ☐	A lot ☐
Are you particularly fussy about keeping your hands clean?	No ☐	A bit ☐	A lot ☐
Do you ever have to do things over and over a certain number of times before they seem quite right?	No ☐	A bit ☐	A lot ☐
Do you ever have trouble finishing your school work or chores because you have to do something over and over again?	No ☐	A bit ☐	A lot ☐
Do you worry a lot if you've done something not exactly the way you like?	No ☐	A bit ☐	A lot ☐
WHEN ANSWERING THE NEXT TWO QUESTIONS, PLEASE THINK OF WHAT WAS MENTIONED IN THE FIRST FIVE QUESTIONS, ESPECIALLY THOSE THAT YOU HAVE ANSWERED 'A lot' OR 'A bit':			
Do these things interfere with your life?	No ☐	A bit ☐	A lot ☐
Do you try to stop them?	No ☐	A bit ☐	A lot ☐

more suggests the need for further assessment for possible obsessive-compulsive disorder; providing the young person is being honest, a score of 5 or less makes obsessive-compulsive disorder unlikely.

After exploring what is going on for the child, internally as well as externally, it is worth exploring **what this means** to him and how he understands what is happening. Some younger children make up interesting stories to make sense of obsessional thoughts – which may sometimes be confused with psychosis. An older child may think he is going mad. Any life stresses or sources of anxiety are likely to be relevant.

Once you have clarified what is going on for the child, and what he will allow you to share with his parents, it may be easier to understand the **parental perspective**. How do they understand what is happening to their child? How do they respond? Do they try to ignore the compulsive behaviours, or do they go along with them? What is the effect on any other family members?

TABLE 39.3 An illustrative diagnostic formulation

	Biological	Psychological	Social
Predisposing (Vulnerability factors)	Holly is an adolescent girl whom boys find attractive There is a family history of anxiety in mother's family	Holly has always been a high achiever, both academically and socially	A year ago, Holly witnessed a man masturbating in the local park, in full view of anyone who passed
Precipitating (Trigger factors)	Holly started her periods six months ago		Boys at school have made lewd comments about Holly, some of which she has overheard
Perpetuating (Maintaining factors)		Counting rituals and going to the toilet reduce Holly's anxiety Holly is afraid she is bad and is going mad, which makes her more anxious	Holly has increasingly avoided social contact, which in turn has made her more socially anxious
Protective (Resilience)		Holly is able to reflect on her thoughts and feelings Holly's parents have realised something must be wrong, and have asked for help promptly	Holly's school teachers are worried about her and would like to help in whatever way they can

BOX 39.3 Alarm Bells in the assessment of OCD

> Compulsions that occupy more than an hour a day
> Obsessions or compulsions that cause the child significant distress
> Significant interference with the child's everyday life, such as home routine, interests, social contact or performance at school

At the end of the history try to arrive at a ***diagnostic formulation*** that considers the predisposing, precipitating and maintaining factors for the child's obsessive-compulsive symptoms (*see* Chapter 6 on Resilience and Risk). An example is shown in Table 39.3, which expands on the case example described above in Box 39.1.

MANAGEMENT AND REFERRAL

Psychoeducation

Begin with an explanation that obsessional thoughts are experienced at least occasionally by almost everyone and that obsessive-compulsive disorder is very common.[7] Those affected may think they are in some way mad, but are definitely *not*. The condition responds well to treatment. Many parents and young people will find some of the information sources mentioned below under 'Resources' helpful, and should be encouraged to join any available local self-help/support groups.

Family support

Explain that obsessive-compulsive disorder is fuelled by anxiety, so anything that raises a child's anxiety may help to maintain the obsessions or compulsions (*see* Figure 39.1 and Table 39.3). Similarly, symptoms may get worse at times of stress or pressure; and any critical comments from family or friends can have the same effect. Don't give the impression that families *cause* obsessive-compulsive disorder, but do emphasise that family members may be able to *help it get better*, for instance by the way they respond to the compulsive behaviours.

Often, parents' attempts to **reassure** their distressed child inadvertently reinforce the anxiety. This is because the child learns to deal with anxiety by getting reassurance from his parents. The reassurance brings only temporary relief, and more expression of anxiety is soon needed to gain repeated reassurance. This becomes a maintaining cycle: the anxiety has to stay bad for the reassurance to keep coming. The way out of this cycle is for the child and parents to become adept at managing the symptoms of obsessive-compulsive disorder, including the associated anxiety: *they must become experts on obsessive-compulsive disorder and unite against it to defeat it together*. Parental strategies that are likely to be more effective than reassurance are shown in Box 39.4.

BOX 39.4 Tips for parents on how to help a child with obsessive-compulsive disorder

Believe your child and respect his point of view. His obsessional thoughts are likely to be real to him (however bizarre or unlikely they may seem to you) and can cause a great deal of distress.

Try not to get embroiled in arguments – for example, whether or not your child's hands are covered in germs – you are unlikely to win.

Try not to get drawn so far into the child's compulsive behaviours that you join in with them.

Try to set time limits to the compulsive behaviours (such as hand-washing): simple statements such as 'That's enough now – it's time to go to school' are likely to be more effective than long discussions.

Try to help your child spot an obsessive thought: noticing an obsession and naming it as such often renders it less distressing and easier to ignore.

Try to help your child ignore his obsessions and associated urges by distracting him with another activity or discussion.

Try to help your child learn how to relax, for example by reading to him, playing a story-tape, getting him to read, playing music to him, getting him to play music, using relaxation tapes or using learnt relaxation routines.

School support

If the child and his parents would like you to, and the obsessive-compulsive disorder is interfering with the child's daily life at school, consider liaising with the school. (Some children, however, show compulsions only at home and not in other contexts.) Encourage the parents to pass on any information they have found helpful to the child's teacher and any other relevant school staff. Some teachers, in common with other professionals, may have preconceived ideas and misconceptions about obsessive-compulsive disorder. It may be helpful to explain the strong link with anxiety and suggest some strategies for responding to compulsions or other expressions of anxiety within school. The community school nurse may be able to play an important part in this.

BOX 39.5 Case Example

Jade is a 10-year-old girl with a moderate learning disability who attends a special school for children with learning difficulties. For a couple months she has been taking other children's pencils from school and bringing them home to her bedroom, where she lines them up and sorts them according to size or colour. She seems to enjoy this immensely, and has hoards of pencils in her room.

Her mother arranges to see a child psychologist, who suggests teaching Jade rules she can understand, such as: 'I must not take things if they are not mine'. Her mother now asks her of anything she does not recognise: 'Is that yours?' This helps a bit, but her tendency to hoard continues.

So Jade's mother and teacher, in discussion with the child psychologist, devise a new strategy. They ensure that the number of pencils Jade has with her are counted out at the beginning and end of each lesson. Her mother uses the same approach whenever she leaves the house, allowing her to take four pencils at a time. At home, when she is on her own in her own room, Jade is allowed to do whatever she likes with her pencils.

Psychological treatment

Cognitive behaviour therapy can be used with children, but has to be adapted to suit the developmental age of the child or young person: behavioural methods are more likely to be effective with younger children and cognitive methods with adolescents who have developed abstract thinking (*see* Chapter 4 on Adolescence). Box 39.5 above shows an example of a purely behavioural intervention, while Box 39.6 below shows how the combined techniques described in the next two paragraphs can be used. Involvement of the child's carers (and possibly other family

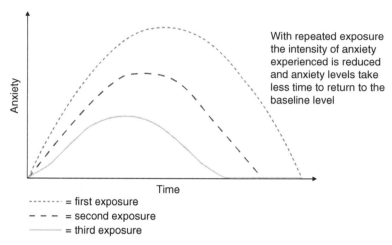

With repeated exposure
the intensity of anxiety
experienced is reduced
and anxiety levels take
less time to return to the
baseline level

------- = first exposure

– – – = second exposure

————— = third exposure

FIGURE 39.2 Anxiety reduction with repeated exposure

members as well) is more likely to be successful than working only with the child in isolation. Initial treatment may be best provided by a primary mental health worker or other Tier 1 or Tier 2 professional, as this may help to de-stigmatise the symptoms. This may be possible only for mild to moderate levels of symptoms: young people with considerable functional impairment, or with significant co-morbid conditions, may need referral to specialist CAMHS.

The two essential components of cognitive behaviour therapy for obsessive-compulsive disorder are *exposure* and *response prevention*. The technique of using ***exposure*** is based upon the finding that anxiety gradually decreases of its own accord after sufficient time face-to-face with the stimulus. In treatment, a young person is encouraged to confront his obsession (and thereby the underlying fear) until the anxiety diminishes. With repeated exposure, the young person learns that nothing really awful will happen – so the obsession loses its power to generate as much anxiety, which therefore decreases. This is shown diagrammatically in Figure 39.2.

Response prevention consists of getting the young person to stop himself from carrying out the compulsions which he has got into the habit of using to reduce his distress. It is important that the young person is on side with this: if he feels this is being forced on him, the process is unlikely to get very far. Preventing covert compulsions (such as silent counting rituals) relies very much on the young person being prepared to reveal what is going on unobserved. Compulsions in younger children commonly involve other people (for instance seeking reassurance), so family members need to be aware of the treatment plan and any role they should have in it.

BOX 39.6 Case Example

John is aged 14 years when his parents become sufficiently concerned about his fear of contamination by germs and repeated hand-washing; they choose to get a referral to the primary mental health worker. John avoids public toilets and will eat only in certain places, as he fears catching a disease from contaminated cutlery or dining room furniture. John describes feeling overwhelmed at times by his fear of contamination. He has become reluctant to go to school, missing some days altogether. He repeatedly asks his parents if they think he has caught a disease and will stop asking them only when they reassure him that he has not.

The primary mental health worker helps John and his family become experts on his symptoms and understand how both his avoidance of what he fears and his parents' repeated reassurance help to maintain his obsessive-compulsive disorder. During the assessment, everyone is encouraged to play detective in identifying all the behaviours that John and his family have evolved to reduce his distress. They then jointly plan a treatment programme involving exposure and response prevention.

In order to explore how this treatment can work for him, John chooses an exposure task he thinks he can manage that they can all try in the clinic room: eating his lunch with cutlery provided from the hospital canteen. They plan this carefully. John identifies the neutralising behaviours he will try to resist: asking his parents for reassurance, not letting his lips touch the fork and brushing his teeth immediately after eating. John agrees to sit out the anxiety arising from this task and wait for it to subside. His parents agree not to reassure him if he asks, but instead to remind him what he has agreed to do.

After 20 minutes of sitting with the food and cutlery in the clinic room, John reports his anxiety starting to feel more tolerable and then dissipating: he is able to place some food in his mouth with the fork and swallow it.

He agrees to repeat the task at home and at school as many times as possible – rating his anxiety each time. John can then see how repeated exposure reduces his anxiety and he is able to resist his compulsions. He goes on to practice what he has learnt in other situations (generalising it) by forcing himself to experience the anxiety (exposure) but without allowing himself to act on it (response prevention). He finds that the anxiety will subside if he is patient enough and works hard enough at telling himself it is going to. The primary mental health worker supports John through these confrontations with his fears, instils optimism, and helps him and his parents see that together they can defeat his obsessive-compulsive disorder.

For a *younger child*, the use of a reward system may help him face up to his anxiety and distress. This can take considerable courage, so any available support should be explored to make it easier to engage in fighting the symptoms. Labelled verbal praise (*see* Chapter 13 on Behaviour Management) from both therapist and parent(s) can encourage progress and help the child see that you recognise and admire the determination he is showing. A child who is unable or unwilling to tackle the problem directly himself may need his parents to expose him gradually, as part of daily family life, to the things he fears.

For some children, *anxiety management techniques* may be very useful (as long as they don't turn into an excuse for avoiding response prevention or an additional compulsion!). For example, using age-appropriate relaxation training or helping the child develop an emotional language to express his feelings (*see* Chapter 20 on Anxiety, Worry, Fears and Phobias).

Cognitive-behavioural techniques can be particularly helpful with young people who are struggling to engage in exposure work. An adolescent with the capacity for self-reflection may benefit from an exploration of how aspects of thinking style can generate anxiety. For example, anxious feelings or obsessions may arise from *cognitive distortions* such as the following.

➤ *Having a mental filter* means focusing on negative consequences such as: 'If the fork touches my lips, I'll get some awful disease' in preference to positive ones such as: 'I've done really well to last 20 minutes with this'.

➤ *Catastrophising* means always thinking the worst will happen, such as believing that if you don't touch the wall seven times before opening the door, you'll have an accident on the way to school.

➤ Having an *exaggerated sense of responsibility* means thinking things are your fault even when they probably aren't. An example is believing that your little sister will come to harm if you don't carry out your counting or touching rituals correctly.

It may be helpful to predict the recurrence of obsessions and compulsions in response to future stresses so as to discuss what techniques have proved most useful and should therefore be tried first next time.

Medication

Medication is not recommended as a first-line treatment for obsessive-compulsive disorder in children and young people, but may be considered by a specialist in Tier 3 CAMHS as a way of reducing the level of anxiety and intensity of obsessional thoughts to a more manageable level, making cognitive-behavioural techniques easier to carry out.

RESOURCES
Websites
Three relevant UK charities are:
- **OCD Action:** www.ocdaction.org.uk
- **OCD-UK:** www.ocduk.org
- **No Panic:** www.nopanic.org.uk

Leaflets
The Royal College of Psychiatrists' factsheets for young people on **obsessive-compulsive disorder and cognitive behaviour therapy are available at:**
- www.rcpsych.ac.uk/mentalhealthinfo/youngpeople/ocd.aspx
- www.rcpsych.ac.uk/mentalhealthinfo/youngpeople/cbt.aspx

From Great Ormond Street Children's Hospital, advice for teachers on how to support young people with obsessive-compulsive disorder in school is available from: www.ich.ucl.ac.uk/gosh_families/information_sheets/obsessive_compulsive_disorder/obsessive_compulsive_disorder_teachers.html

Books for young people and their parents

- Chansky TE. *Freeing Your Child from Obsessive-Compulsive Disorder*. New York, NY: Times Books; 2001.
- Wagner AP. *Up and Down the Worry Hill: a children's book about obsessive-compulsive disorder and its treatment*. Rochester, NY: Lighthouse Press; 2004.
- Wagner AP. *What to Do When Your Child Has Obsessive-Compulsive Disorder: Strategies and solutions*. Rochester, NY: Lighthouse Press; 2002.
- Wells J. *Touch and Go Jo: an adolescent's experience of OCD*. London: Jessica Kingsley; 2006. The story of one teenager's battle against obsessive-compulsive disorder, this contains information and helpful tips.
- Wever C, Phillips N. *The Secret Problem*. New South Wales: Shrink-Rap Press (Australia). A book with clear and simple text and drawings to bring the symptoms and solutions to life. Available from: www.shrinkrap.com.au

Books for professionals

- Wagner AP. *Treatment of OCD in Children and Adolescents: a cognitive-behaviour therapy manual*. Rochester, NY: Lighthouse Press; 2003.
- Stallard P. *Think Good – Feel Good: a cognitive behaviour therapy workbook for children and young people*. Chichester and Oxford: Wiley-Blackwell; 2002.
- Stallard P. *A Clinician's Guide to Think Good, Feel Good: using CBT with children and young people*. Chichester and Oxford: Wiley-Blackwell; 2005.

REFERENCES

1 National Institute for Health and Clinical Excellence. *Obsessive-compulsive Disorder (OCD) and Body Dysmorphic Disorder (BDD): core interventions in the treatment of obsessive-compulsive disorder and body dysmorphic disorder* [NICE Clinical Guidance 31]. London: NICE; 2005. Available at: http://guidance.nice.org.uk/CG31 (accessed 5 April 2011).
2 Carr A. *The Handbook of Child & Adolescent Clinical Psychology*. Routledge: London; 1999.
3 Ibid.
4 Rachman S, Hodgson R. *Obsessions and Compulsions*. New Jersey: Prentice-Hall; 1980.
5 Bolton D, Luckie M, Steinberg D. Long-term course of obsessive-compulsive disorder treated in adolescence. *Journal of the American Academy of Child and Adolescent Psychiatry*. 1995; **32**(11): 1441–50.
6 Uher R, Heyman I, Mortimore C, *et al.* Screening young people for obsessive compulsive disorder. *BJP.* 2007; **191**: 353–4. The Short Obsessive Compulsive Screener (SOCS) can be downloaded from: http://ocdyouth.iop.kcl.ac.uk/downloads/socs.pdf (accessed 5 April 2011).
7 Carr, op. cit.

CHAPTER 40

Recurrent abdominal pain

INTRODUCTION

Recurrent abdominal pain can be defined as the occurrence of at least three episodes of pain interfering with normal activities in a three-month period. This is a common problem in school-age children, and it is likely that every child experiences tummy pain at some stage. Estimates of **prevalence** vary, partly because many suffer in silence and partly because of unresolved debates about definitions: an early estimate was 10%, but this has been revised upwards to 11–45%.[1,2,3] Boys and girls are similarly affected and there is no clear social class disparity.

Many affected children may be diagnosed as suffering from a condition with a name that may be more acceptable to parents, such as irritable bowel syndrome or abdominal migraine. Many have some **other physical symptoms**, such as pain elsewhere (often headaches), gut complaints, or chronic-fatigue-like symptoms such as fatigue, dizziness, numbness or weakness. The experience of tummy pain itself may be partly due to increased awareness or sensitivity to that sort of pain: visceral hyperalgesia.[4] Affected children may be more likely to perceive physical symptoms as threatening; more likely to have symptoms of **anxiety** or depression; more likely to have suffered some adverse life-events; more likely to find life challenges overwhelming; and more likely to experience anxiety in the future.[5,6,7]

A child whose parent takes her to a professional (probably most often the family's general practitioner) usually has some **functional impairment**, such as a reduction in school attendance, social life or other activities. Presentation to a helping professional may result from concerns of school staff. Parents may fear that the child has a serious illness that has not yet been diagnosed, and may therefore justifiably seek referral to a paediatrician. When paediatric assessment does not show an identifiable explanation for the pain, the child is more likely to recover if parents can accept that there may be other ways of understanding at least the persistence of the symptoms.[8]

ASSESSMENT

Engagement

It is all too easy to get off to a bad start with the parents of a child who repeatedly complains of tummy pain and the child herself, for instance by giving the impression that you think it is somehow not real or is 'all in her mind' (even without saying any of these words). It is essential:

> to acknowledge the child's suffering
> to emphasise that you believe the child when she talks about the pain
> to acknowledge the family's concerns about what the pain may mean
> *not* to challenge the reality of the symptoms
> *not* to prejudge the cause: a 'don't know' attitude is probably safer.

History of the pain

If the child has not yet seen a paediatrician, it is worth exploring *the nature of the pain* in some depth. Try to obtain a clear description of what the pain feels like, where it is, and when it occurs. Establish if there are any patterns to the pain: for instance, does it occur more in school time or in advance of particular activities?

TABLE 40.1 Aspects of tummy pain worth asking about

Worrying	Not so worrying
Age less than five years	Age five years or more
Acute onset	Vague onset
Continuous	Intermittent/recurrent
Well-localised	Poorly localised
May radiate to the back	Central without radiation
Peripheral (Apley's law)	The child points at or near the umbilicus
One pain only	Aches or pains occur elsewhere in the body, a common example being a headache
Joint pains	No joint pains
Wakes the child at night	The child is not woken by the pain
Diminished appetite, weight loss or delayed growth	The child eats well and is growing satisfactorily
Fever	No fever
Rash(es)	No rash
Vomiting – particularly if bilious	Nausea at most
Urinary symptoms such as frequency or pain	No urinary symptoms of concern
Bowel symptoms such as hard poo, infrequent poos, runny poo, frequent poos or blood in poo	No bowel symptoms of concern
Pain associated with monthly cycle or heavy menstrual bleeding	Boy, premenstrual girl, or pain unrelated to periods
No relation to school day	Occurs on school mornings only
No evidence of emotional distress	Evidence of anxiety, salient life events or unhappiness
Family history of inflammatory bowel disease Crohn's, ulcerative colitis, or liver disease	No family history of tummy symptoms

Has the child found that the pain enables her to avoid certain situations or people? Ask the questions indicated in Table 40.1. If there are significant symptoms in the left-hand column, consider arranging a paediatric assessment. This may lead to a diagnosis for instance of abdominal migraine, irritable bowel syndrome or constipation.

Establish a picture of how the child is managing *day-to-day life* and the family's usual activities: this may reveal unexpected symptoms. For example, an adolescent with abdominal pain may disclose, on detailed questioning, reduced eating and increased exercise, which suggests the possibility of an eating disorder – not at first suspected. Asking the child or family the question 'If the tummy pain had a voice, what would it be saying?' may reveal information you have not considered (such as child abuse).

Family and social history

A brief *family history* is important, including if time a family tree. This should reveal any relevant illnesses in family members. It is important not just to ask about illnesses in the family but also to ask about how those illnesses impact on the family. It is common for a parent to have irritable bowel syndrome, migraine, anxiety or depression.[9] Do the parents or the child have particular concern about an underlying cause of tummy pain that has occurred in a friend or family member?

BOX 40.1 Case Example

> It is not until she helps construct a family tree that eight-year-old Christine discloses that her great-aunt Ada died about a year ago of stomach cancer. Ada's first symptom was tummy pain, which her doctor did not initially think was at all serious.

The family history can lead on to a discussion of any relevant *life events*. Examples include: bereavement, changes in peer relationships (such as a best friend moving away), moving school or house, stresses at school (such as bullying or not getting on with a teacher) or illness in a family member.

The discussion so far may reveal whether the child becomes easily stressed or anxious. It is worth asking specifically about symptoms of *anxiety or depression*.

To expand on your understanding of the pain, obtain permission to ask for *information from other sources*, such as school or club leaders.

Management

Try not to get too tied in knots about the difference between 'organic' and 'non-organic' causes of abdominal pain. It is likely to be more helpful to emphasise the inseparability of physical and psychological features in many paediatric conditions. For instance, any pain is worrying, as it may have a serious cause. The child is likely to be more worried if surrounding adults are. Worrying about the pain will give it centre stage, and make it feel worse than if it can be allotted a minor role. Anxiety about the pain can have physical components, such as 'butterflies in the tummy', which can contribute to the experience of pain in a positive feedback loop (vicious circle). Ignoring the pain or at least learning to live with it may be a more realistic goal than a complete 'cure'. Interim goals should be steadily achievable, such as gradually optimising school attendance, social contacts or physical activities.

It is essential to form a collaborative relationship with parents, who should be encouraged to see themselves as part coach (encouraging progress towards goals) and part protector (avoiding, within reason, situations that make the pain worse). Passivity, avoidance and wishful thinking can make the pain more difficult to deal with, whereas actively trying to cope with the pain and adjust to it can make it more tolerable. Emphasise the child's strength in withstanding the pain and competence in working out how best to deal with it. Join with the parents and child in fighting against whatever impact the pain has.

Specific strategies that may help include the following.

➤ Assuming that serious illness has been excluded, explain that although the pain is real it is not a sign of a serious illness and that *the child will recover* from each episode.

➤ *Psychoeducation* could include an emphasis on the reality of the pain and the associated suffering, but suggest that the way we react to pain differs. Some people may perceive pain as a threat that can disable them; others may find ways of tolerating it and getting on with things, *despite* the pain.

➤ Negotiate *goals* with which the child and parents feel comfortable, and which are achievable and emphasise *coping with* rather than *curing*.

➤ Explore with the child and parents any times when she does *not* have the pain and note these *exceptions* – so as to build on them.

➤ Help the child and family to identify *diversion strategies* that help distract the child from the pain such as: playing with friends, any enjoyable form of exercise, or joint family activities.

➤ Encourage parents to *give as little attention as possible to the pain* – and in particular to avoid repeated reassurance; they can use the diversionary strategies identified.

➤ Help the child and family identify *ways of managing* the pain or lessening it, such as: a warm hot water bottle at bedtime, a tummy massage, a particular hot drink.

➤ *Dietary approaches* may also help, involving if necessary a paediatric dietician. If dietary triggers can be identified, it is worth doing a trial of avoiding specific foods for a period of time. It is probably sensible to recommend regular meals including adequate fruit, vegetables, fibre and fluids. Increasing the fibre content of the diet may help reduce the frequency of pain attacks.[10]

➤ Building plenty of physical exercise into the child's daily routine is likely to help, using a graded approach as in chronic fatigue syndrome (*see* Chapter 29).[11] Involving a paediatric physiotherapist may help with this process.

➤ Encourage the child to attend *school* or activities as normal whilst acknowledging she may feel the pain more at these times.

➤ Explain the analogy of how sometimes people can feel 'sick with worry' in order to introduce the idea of an *emotional component* to the pain.

➤ Encourage the child to share any worries with someone they can trust such as a parent or teacher so that *stressors* can be dealt with in the open, rather than niggling away without being spoken about.

➤ If identifiable stressors emerge, such as bullying or specific learning difficulty, these should be dealt with, using a joint *problem-solving* approach, involving school staff if appropriate.

➤ If *life events* seem to play an important part, then it may help to schedule time for the child to talk to someone about these (you or someone else).

➤ The role of *medication* is debatable: professional support with the above coping strategies is preferable, if available. The problem with a painkiller such as ibuprofen is that it may irritate the lining of the stomach. Peppermint oil has been shown to help in irritable bowel syndrome[12] and pizotifen in abdominal migraine.[13] Citalopram has also shown potential.[14]

BOX 40.2 Case Example

Due to several bouts of tummy pain, nine-year-old Aaron repeatedly misses several consecutive days of school. After several visits to the health centre, his general practitioner refers him to a hospital paediatrician.

The paediatrician takes a history, does a thorough examination and does some basic investigations, including routine blood tests, a urine culture and an abdominal ultrasound. There is nothing in any of the results of these tests to confirm Aaron's parents' fear that something serious underlies his pain.

When they meet with the paediatrician to discuss the test results, Aaron's parents reflect that the pain has been worse during term-times and seems not so much of a problem during the school holidays. They agree to meet with the paediatric liaison nurse (who works one day per week in paediatrics and the other four days in specialist CAMHS) to discuss how best to manage Aaron's pain.

At her first meeting with Aaron and his parents, the paediatric liaison nurse acknowledges how real Aaron's pain is and the effects it is having on his life and activities. She explains that she hopes together they will be able to find ways he can cope with his pain so that his everyday life will become less disrupted.

She discovers during her own reassessment that Aaron is far more likely to have the pain at the beginning than end of the week. His parents acknowledge that he is an anxious child at times but they are not aware of any difficulties at school, and Aaron does not volunteer any.

The paediatric liaison nurse meets with Aaron and his parents for four sessions, at roughly fortnightly intervals. They discuss strategies to help Aaron cope with the pain, such as finding things that will distract him and learning to keep going with his daily routine in spite of the pain. She explains the way in which anxiety (about the pain or about anything else) can augment the pain, and teaches Aaron and his mother some anxiety management strategies (*see* Chapter 20 on Anxiety, Worry, Fears and Phobias). She persuades Aaron to notice the times when he does not have pain rather than the times when he does.

The paediatric liaison nurse encourages Aaron's parents to be positive and calm with their son, to enable him to get to school – even on days when his pain is at its worst. With the family's permission, she discusses Aaron's difficulties with his class teacher to include the school in the management plan. The head teacher allocates a support worker with whom Aaron can spend time if he feels unwell: he is given a card to show the class teacher when he feels things are too much for him, and then he is allowed to go to the school library until the next lesson. His support worker joins him in the library when she is free, and helps him return to the class as soon as he feels ready. The paediatric liaison nurse also makes the community school nurse aware of the situation so she can monitor progress with school staff and subsequently take over follow-up support with the family

If the pain comes on at home, Aaron has worked out that he can relax by watching a favourite DVD, playing a game with one or both of his parents, or going to the nearby playground with a neighbour of his.

The paediatric liaison nurse gets Aaron to rate his pain and its impact on 10-point scales, with 10 being the worst. Initially, the score during bouts of pain goes up to 9/10 and the score for overall impact is 8/10. Although the score for pain sensation during bouts goes down only to 7/10, the impact score gradually decreases over the course of the four sessions to a 3/10. Aaron learns to go into school even if he has tummy pain in the mornings; he becomes increasingly confident that this will wear off over the course of the day.

Aaron's ability to cope with his pain is so much better after four sessions – it is less frequent but almost as severe when it comes – that his parents agree with the paediatric liaison nurse that they do not need any more appointments with her, but will instead keep in contact with the community school nurse. She does a home visit, then monitors the situation at school and contacts Aaron's mother by telephone if necessary. After a follow-up appointment, the paediatrician discharges Aaron form her clinic.

REFERRAL

Involvement of a paediatrician should be arranged at an early stage if there is any doubt at all about the significance of the child's symptoms. Involvement of specialist CAMHS may be necessary (preferably after paediatric assessment) if there is no paediatric liaison or primary child and adolescent mental health service or equivalent. Some parents may not want involvement of any mental health professional, in which case a member of the paediatric or primary care team will need to take on the tasks described in this chapter.

BOX 40.3 Practice Points for recurrent abdominal pain

Always acknowledge to the child and family that the pain is real.

Take a clear history of the pain and any related family and social factors. If this suggests worrying symptoms, refer to a paediatrician (if this has not already been done).

Identify with the family ways of coping with the pain that keep to a minimum the pain's interference in the child's day-to-day life.

REFERENCES

1 Christensen MF. Rome II Classification—the final delimitation of functional abdominal pains in children? *J Pediatr Gastroenterol Nutr.* 2004; **39**(3): 303–4.

2 Apley J, Naish N. Recurrent abdominal pains: a field survey of 1,000 school children. Arch Dis Child. 1958; **33**(168): 165–70.

3 Plunkett A, Beattie RM. Recurrent abdominal pain in childhood. *J R Soc Med.* 2005; **98**(3): 101–6.

4 Di Lorenzo C, Youssef NN, Sigurdsson L, *et al.* Visceral hyperalgesia in children with functional abdominal pain. *J Pediatr.* 2001; **139**(6): 838–43.

5 Campo JV, Di Lorenzo C, Chiappetta L, *et al.* Adult outcomes of pediatric recurrent abdominal pain: do they just grow out of it? *Pediatrics.* 2001; **108**(1): E1.

6 Campo JV, Bridge J, Ehmann M, *et al.* Recurrent abdominal pain, anxiety, and depression in primary care. *Pediatrics.* 2004; **113**(4): 817–24.

7 Campo, 2001, op. cit.

8 Crushell E, Rowland M, Doherty M, *et al.* Importance of parental conceptual model of illness in severe recurrent abdominal pain. Pediatrics. 2003; **112**(6 Pt 1): 1368–72.

9 Campo JV, Bridge J, Lucas A, *et al.* Physical and emotional health of mothers of youth with functional abdominal pain. *Archives of Pediatrics & Adolescent Medicine.* 2007; **161**(2): 131–7.

10 Paulo AZ, Amancio OM, de Morais MB, *et al.* Low-dietary fiber intake as a risk factor for recurrent abdominal pain in children. *EJCN.* 2006; **60**(7): 823–7.

11 Plunkett, op. cit.

12 Kline RM, Kline JJ, DiPalma J, *et al.* Enteric coated, pH dependent peppermint oil capsules for the treatment of irritable bowel syndrome in children. *J Pediatr.* 2001; **138**(1): 125–8.

13 Symon DNK, Russell G. Double blind placebo controlled trial of pizotifen syrup in the treatment of abdominal migraine. *Arch Dis Child.* 1995; **72**(1): 48–50.

14 Campo JV, Perel J, Lucas A, *et al.* Citalopram treatment of pediatric recurrent abdominal pain and comorbid internalizing disorders: an exploratory study. *J Am Acad Child Adolesc Psychiatry.* 2004; **43**(10): 1234–42.

Physical presentations of emotional distress

INTRODUCTION

Up to 5% of children consulting general practitioners have a primary mental health problem.[1] Considering broader psychosocial factors that may have some relevance raises this figure to 20% of children who present to a professional with a physical complaint.[2,3] Emotional distress can present itself in a number of ways and can be expressed in the form of very real physical symptoms: these are in no sense imaginary.

➤ Anxiety can lead to (or consist of) physical symptoms such as a fast heart rate, chest pain, shakiness, sweating, shortness of breath, a dry mouth, tummy pain, diarrhoea, dizziness, pins and needles and pallor (going pale) – *see* Table 20.1 in Chapter 20 on Anxiety, Worry, Fears and Phobias.

➤ Headaches can often be a manifestation of tension or distress. Recurrent headaches and abdominal pain are a very common way for emotional factors to present in childhood.

➤ Some physical conditions that are intrinsically painful may give rise to anticipatory anxiety that may take the same form as the physical pain – or at least worsen it. An example could be the pain due to a bone tumour that is exacerbated by thoughts about what the tumour is going to do. Another parallel example is the anticipatory vomiting that can occur *before* the injection of a cancer chemotherapy agent that reliably causes vomiting.

➤ Physical complaints may occur without discernible organic cause: a common example being recurrent abdominal pain. However, sometimes a cause may eventually be found for such symptoms, such as abdominal migraine in the case of tummy pain, so it behoves professionals to keep an open mind. And even without an identifiable physical cause, it is important not to fall into the trap of thinking that the symptom is 'all in the mind' or in some way fabricated or unreal. Even if the symptom is 'only' due to an otherwise unexpressed emotion, this does not make it any the less real – pain is no less painful whatever the cause.

Thorough assessment is important to ensure that both emotional and physical dimensions of the presenting problem are understood as well as possible. It is as dangerous to miss an emotional crisis such as sexual abuse as it is to miss a surgical crisis such as appendicitis. As a number of different terms are used to describe overlapping physical and emotional conditions, some definitions may be helpful.

Terminology

A physical presentation of emotional distress is any physical presentation where the doctor feels that psychological or social factors are contributing in a significant way. An example would be asthma where some form of stress seems to be contributing.

Somatisation is a narrower term used to describe the way that some physical symptoms are especially likely to represent emotional distress (such as tummy pains and headaches). For a diagrammatic representation of this as a spectrum, see Figure 41.1. In these cases, the child (or parent) is likely to complain of a physical problem and both are likely to want an acceptable diagnosis and treatment. It may not be acceptable for a professional to use the term 'somatisation', as this may be interpreted as implying that the symptom is not 'real'.

Hysteria has been defined as the presence of physical symptoms in the absence of disease, or where the disease is present but insufficient to explain the symptom. An alternative way to look at hysteria is as *abnormal illness behaviour*. By taking on the sick role, the child may be gaining a number of advantages such as:

➤ more attention from parents
➤ not having to separate from parents
➤ reduced conflict at home
➤ permission not to attend school
➤ an opt-out from expected high achievement
➤ additional support
➤ attention from multiple professionals.

The term 'hysteria' has gone out of favour because it has been used in so many senses, some derogatory. The concept of '*conversion disorder*' derives from the Freudian idea that an internal conflict, usually unconscious, manifests externally as ('converts' to) a physical symptom. This symptom cannot be explained by known pathological mechanisms. Absence of a physical explanation is a dangerous criterion to use on its own: long-term follow-up studies have shown that up to 50% of so-called 'hysterical disorders' turn out to be a rare condition that the clinician hadn't thought of, didn't know about or couldn't detect.[4]

Dissociation is discussed in Chapter 37 on adjustment disorder and post-traumatic stress disorder as a mode of self-protection that involves *not* remembering something traumatic or painful that it may feel safer not to think about. Because the feelings associated with this past experience are still lurking somewhere, they may be expressed in various indirect ways, one of which is in

Completely	Completely
somatic	psychological

FIGURE 41.1 The spectrum of childhood illness

the form of physical symptoms. If so, 'dissociative disorder' may look the same as 'conversion disorder': the young person *dissociates* from the horrific unconscious memories, which are *converted* to a physical symptom that may be safer, but is otherwise inexplicable.

The term '***secondary gain***' also derives from Freudian ideas. The *primary* gain consists of not having to deal consciously with whatever conflicts or unpleasant memories are converted into physical symptoms. The *secondary* gain consists of the (perhaps unexpected) rewards of this such as the seven bullet points mentioned above under 'abnormal illness behaviour'.

Family factors may also be relevant: for example, some children find that their parents will agree with each other only when the child is ill. Such significant advantages of illness behaviour can also be regarded as ***functions*** of the symptom(s). This way of looking at unexplained symptoms does *not* imply conscious intent, manipulation or fabrication. The rewards of being ill can also be seen as maintaining or perpetuating causes (*see* Table 6.3 in Chapter 6 on Resilience and Risk).

It may be worth adding a comment here on the word ***manipulative***, which is sometimes used to describe a young person. It is important to be clear with parents and other professionals that the symptoms are likely to serve an important function for the child and this is what needs to be explored. To describe the child as being manipulative implies purposeful behaviour and is simply unhelpful to understanding her situation and managing it. There may be rare occasions when the child is consciously aware of getting her own way by exaggerating her symptoms: even then, it is more important to be curious about what makes the child need to do this than to dismiss her actions with a pejorative label.

BOX 41.1 Case Example

Virginia, aged 10 years, complains of tummy pain that comes on frequently. It gets so bad that her general practitioner refers her to hospital, and the hospital paediatrician is pressurised by Virginia's mother to admit her for observation. This admission helps to suggest that there is no serious origin to the pain.

Virginia has an older sister who has had a bone marrow transplant for acute myeloid leukaemia and multiple hospital admissions. Their mother is able to agree with ward staff that Virginia has missed out on parental attention as a result.

Fabricated or induced illness is something quite different from any of the above, and is discussed in Chapter 12 on Child Abuse and Safeguarding. It is mentioned here because it could be regarded as a child's physical expression of a parent's emotional distress.

ASSESSMENT

A clear ***history*** of the presenting problems needs to be taken from the child and the carers. Ideally, this should include the professional spending individual time with the child and parents separately so that each can freely discuss any concerns. Younger children may find it easier to put difficult feelings into a picture.

Examples of the way in which the child's emotional distress may present as physical symptoms include the following:

➤ tension headaches

➤ recurrent abdominal pain (*see* Chapter 40)

➤ asthma attacks brought on by anxiety or associated with hyperventilation

➤ diarrhoea or constipation related to anxiety

➤ vomiting

➤ autonomic nervous symptoms that can occur as an expression of anxiety, as listed above

➤ pseudo-convulsions – these often occur in children who already have epilepsy and so are familiar with fits and the likely professional reaction to them

➤ deficit symptoms: aphasia, loss of vision, loss of hearing, loss of sensation that is not consistent with the anatomy of sensory nerve supply or weakness in a pattern that is not consistent with the anatomy of motor nerve supply

➤ active symptoms: abnormal movements, or pain that is not consistent with the anatomy of sensory nerve supply

➤ poor sleep pattern leading to being too tired to attend school

➤ the child being excessively disabled in comparison to the objective effects of the disease. Occasionally, a child will suffer from a genuine physical illness but the symptoms will persist when the organic cause has resolved. Sometimes, disabling symptoms seem to have started with a minor physical illness such as a cold.

As well as a history of the physical symptoms it is important to find out if the family has suffered any *stress* during or before the illness, for instance bullying or a change in family circumstances.

It is also useful to find out the *impact* of the illness on the child and the family. For instance, has the child had to take time off school or has a carer had to stay off work to look after her?

Examination may show inconsistencies between the nature of the symptoms and neuroanatomy. *Observation* may show inexplicable changes in symptoms over time. *Investigations* such as blood tests and scans should be kept to a minimum.

It is important to convince the child and parent that you are taking each seriously even though you feel the cause of the physical symptoms may be mainly psychological in nature.

For some children, the situation remains unclear after a single assessment. They may therefore require an extended assessment over time. This may take the form of repeated direct observations, perhaps using a symptom record. For instance, for a child reporting pain it may be helpful for her to fill in at regular intervals a pain scale (which could be a sequence of faces with different expressions for younger children or a 10 cm line for adolescents). These observations or measures can help identify any patterns in the symptoms or any factors that ameliorate or worsen them.

MANAGEMENT

If the family acknowledges the possibility of a psychological cause for the problem, treatment is much easier. Some parents are open to the suggestion that stress or emotional distress may have a part to play in their child's illness, especially if you show that you are taking the symptoms seriously. Explanations that having such symptoms may be very stressful or distressing, and that in some children stress or psychological upsets can make physical symptoms worse, can often help the engagement of the child and family in co-operation with professionals.

If the family accept that (di)stress is a component of the problem, then education about the nature of anxiety, its symptoms and advice about anxiety management can be introduced (*see* Chapter 20 on Anxiety, Worry, Fears and Phobias). The child and parents can be actively involved in this process, helping to set their own goals for return to full health. Treatment may include diary-keeping, symptom measures, ratings of anxiety, positive self-statements, and exercises in relaxation or breathing. It is important, however, to be clear with the family that the child's experience is very real and her symptoms are genuine, even if no organic cause can be found and even though (di)stress may be playing a part in the symptoms. Be vigilant about saying you believe in the symptoms even if you don't: the child will not return to you if she thinks you don't believe her. It is important to follow such children up and monitor their progress.

Suggestion can be helpful with these children. A good prognosis should be given at an early stage, with the advice that recovery should occur quickly. This is a particularly important strategy for professionals in a position of authority, such as for instance a consultant paediatrician or paediatric neurologist: the predicted timescale for the resolution of symptoms can become fixed in the minds of family members.

The difficulty for many children is how to relinquish the symptoms without *loss of face*. Strategies to manage the symptoms whilst minimising the impact on everyday activities should be encouraged, for instance encouraging and praising daily attendance at school despite headaches. One particularly successful face-saving treatment may be a course of physiotherapy.

Members of the primary care team who can offer ongoing support include the general practitioner, practice nurse, community school nurse, pastoral care workers in schools, school counsellors, teachers, Connexions workers, family link workers and primary mental health workers. Members of the hospital team who may help include not only the consultant paediatrician, but also the paediatric physiotherapist, occupational therapist or youth worker. A team around the child may form, in which case a meeting for professionals and family may help to coordinate the support for the child.

REFERRAL

Referral to a paediatrician should be made early if the situation is at all complicated or if there is a question about the diagnosis. For simpler problems, referral should be considered if the symptoms do not improve appreciably within about a month to six weeks. An onward referral for joint working with specialist CAMHS can then be made by the paediatrician if she feels this is warranted and providing that the family are able to accept such a referral.

Some families will refer themselves to alternative therapists, with positive results, particularly if this is the normal practice for the family if someone is unwell.

BOX 41.2 Case Example

Sophie, aged 13 years, is referred to the hospital paediatrician by her general practitioner with persistent episodes of vomiting. At the assessment, it becomes clear that there is in fact frequent nausea but very little vomiting. Due to the symptoms, Sophie is missing a lot of school, as she tends to feel sick in the mornings and then stays home for the day. Sophie's mother acknowledges that Sophie is a sensitive girl who often worries about things. The paediatrician acknowledges that Sophie is suffering from a lot of nausea and asks if the family would be prepared to meet with a primary mental health worker (together with him) to look at managing the stress caused by the problem. The paediatrician also prescribes domperidone 10–20 mg three times a day before meals for the nausea and says that he will need to continue to review Sophie regularly.

Sophie and her mother meet with the primary mental health worker and discuss how the illness is impacting Sophie's life. The main area appears to be school attendance and after-school clubs. Sophie is encouraged to go to school even on the days she feels sick and even if she ends up being in school a little late on those days. The primary mental health worker agrees to liaise with the school to ensure that school staff will be tolerant towards Sophie's potential late arrival. She also speaks with the school welfare assistant, who agrees that Sophie can have the option of visiting her, and if necessary staying for a brief period in the sick room, if the nausea seems unmanageable. Sophie agrees to keep a diary of her attendance at school and meets regularly with the primary mental health worker over the next two months and less regularly over the following six months.

Over this period, Sophie initially visits the school welfare assistant two to three times a week, but then appears to settle and visit less often. She needs a lot of reassurance that she is managing her symptoms well. There is a gradual improvement in Sophie's attendance in school. She also eventually rejoins an after-school dance class. She continues to complain of some nausea, but there are no episodes of vomiting. She also continues to be reviewed every two months by the paediatrician over the next eight months. She is then offered a six-monthly review with the option to return sooner if she needs to. After a further six months, she and her mother are able to accept being discharged.

BOX 41.3 Practice Points for physical presentations of emotional distress

Keep an open mind about the origin of any symptoms.

Believe in the distress: convince the child and parent(s) that you believe the symptoms are real.

Try to find a face-saving way for the child to return to normal functioning (such as physiotherapy, or increasing school attendance very gradually).

Predict that the symptoms will subside.

Predict a quick resolution if you feel able to.

Refer to a paediatrician if:

- there is doubt about the diagnosis
- the family requires a specialist opinion
- it looks as if the problem may become intractable.

REFERENCES

1 Garralda ME, Bailey D. Children with psychiatric disorders in primary care. *Journal of Child Psychology and Psychiatry.* 1986; **27**(5): 611–24. Epub 7 Dec 2006.
2 Bailey V, Graham P, Boniface D. How much child psychiatry does a general practitioner do? *J R Coll Gen Pract.* 1978; **28**: 621–6.
3 Garralda ME. Primary care psychiatry. In: Rutter M, Taylor E, Hersov L. *Child and Adolescent Psychiatry.* Oxford: Blackwell; 1994. pp. 1055–70.
4 Marsden CD. Hysteria: a neurologist's view. *Psychological Medicine.* 1986; **16**(2): 277–88.

CHAPTER 42

Chronic paediatric illness[1]

INTRODUCTION

Acute illness may be a shock that has a reverberating impact on any family. Resilient children and families are likely to return, after a limited period, to normal functioning and their usual routine – providing recovery is complete. In contrast, the consequences of a *continuing (chronic) illness* permeate every aspect of the child's life, and are likely to affect every member of the family to some extent. It is normal for chronic illness to have significant psychological and social consequences, but that does not make these effects any easier to deal with. The nature of the consequences will depend on a number of factors, such as the following.

➤ The *age of onset* – A child who develops a chronic illness after being completely well will follow a different path, and have a different impact on other family members, from a child who is born with a health problem or disability that persists.

➤ The **stage of development:**
  — *life stage* – a child who is just starting school will experience a different impact from an adolescent who is already beginning to exercise a degree of independence
  — *level of understanding* – It may be very difficult to explain to a toddler what has to be done. An older child should be able to understand enough to accept what is going on, providing everything possible is explained at an age-appropriate level.

➤ The *outcome* **of the condition** – Parents may react completely differently if they feel their child is unlikely to survive. An expected demise in late adolescence or early adulthood from muscular dystrophy or cystic fibrosis is more complicated to deal with than the intermittent reminders of impairment in diabetes or severe asthma. Cancer may create issues different from either of these, in that the outcome may be uncertain for much of the duration of the illness, and 'cure' may be associated with adverse consequences such as short stature, infertility, disfigurement, continuing medication or the risk of a second cancer.

➤ The *nature of the disability* – Multiple congenital anomalies have a different impact from recurrent diabetic ketoacidosis.

➤ The *extent of the disability* – Most children would experience a greater impact from being wheelchair-bound due to muscular dystrophy than from living with a false leg after an amputation for a bone tumour.

➤ The child's *resilience* and family's coping style – Some children and their families are more able to cope with adversity, and bounce back, than others.

➤ The family's *support* mechanisms – Severe chronic illness can put a major strain on marital and other family relationships, often leading to the emergence of unexpected strengths and resources.

— The family's *cultural and religious beliefs* and ability to change and adapt – Is a chronic illness an ordeal or an opportunity? Some families may see illness as a random event; others as a punishment; others as an opportunity to learn and develop or re-organise how they function.

ASSESSMENT

It may be useful to think about the effects on different family members, on the family as a whole and on non-family members. One way of approaching this is to consider first the effects on the child, then the effects on the parents, then on other family members living at home, then on family members elsewhere, and lastly (but not least) on the child's friends.

The effects on the *child* may include the following.

➤ *A disturbance of self-image* – The young person may feel different in a variety of ways. Self-esteem may be affected, sometimes to the extent of depression. Some children express their negative feelings about themselves in behavioural disturbance. Bodily deformations are particularly difficult to tolerate in adolescence, when identity is developing. Illnesses that do not show on the outside may still lead to feelings such as 'Why me?'

➤ *Relationships with peers* – Opportunities for social activities may be reduced. For instance, a young person with diabetes may not be able to go to a sleepover because a friend's parents may be scared of the illness, or not be allowed to go for a long walk with friends for fear of a hypoglycaemic attack.

➤ *Bullying* (*see* Chapter 22) – Clinical experience and research both indicate that a young person with any chronic illness is more likely to be bullied.[2]

➤ *Disruption of school* – School attendance may be reduced because of recurrent hospital admissions, such as in leukaemia or severe asthma, or by exhaustion, as in chronic fatigue syndrome. School performance may be affected by cognitive impairment, as in leukaemia; by physical limitations, as in asthma; or by the emotional distractions of being ill. This can reinforce feelings of being different or not fitting in and make it harder to sustain close friendships.

➤ *Dislike of treatment* – Children with cystic fibrosis may get fed up with repeated physiotherapy, or having to ingest large quantities of pancreatic enzymes at every meal. Children with leukaemia may dread their visits to hospital, where injections cause vomiting, and some treatments may require prolonged social isolation. Some children learn to vomit at the thought of an injection; others may develop procedural anxiety, which can make routine blood tests and drips an ordeal for everyone.

➤ *Poor adherence* (which used to be called compliance) – Whether because of the side effects of treatment, the implication that she is different, or just the gnawing boredom of having to take medication every day, a young person with a chronic illness is likely to go through periods of not wanting to adhere to recommended treatment (and not necessarily tell anyone about it).

Effects on *parents* include the following.

➤ *Bereavement* **for the loss of the perfect child** – Parents may go through the well-described stages of reaction to being told their child has a chronic illness: denial, anger, guilt, bargaining and finally acceptance (*see* Chapter 10 on Death, Dying and Bereavement). But they need not necessarily experience these stages at the same time – which may reduce the support they can give to each other. Going through some or all of these stages may happen more than once: not only at initial diagnosis but also subsequently at key transitions in a child's life, such as: changing school, leaving school, starting work, leaving home, and having children of his own.

BOX 42.1 Case Example

> Eustace has a severe chronic illness to which his parents have reacted in opposite ways. His mother is very involved in supporting him through all the tests and treatments, whereas his father acts as if there is nothing much wrong with his son, leaving all the 'medical stuff' to his wife. This makes it difficult for them to support each other: father feels left out and mother feels unappreciated.

➤ *Chronic sorrow*, because the child continues to be less than perfect. This could be seen as a long, drawn-out bereavement reaction. Particularly with significant handicap, there may be new effects emerging at different ages, and as the child becomes older, the differences from other children become more and more starkly apparent.

➤ *Over-protectiveness* – It is too easy to be critical of an overprotective parent; it is in general difficult to tell how much a concerned and restrictive attitude arises from the parent's personality, and how much from the risky nature of the illness. Health professionals can easily forget that many common illnesses such as asthma and epilepsy are life-threatening, and deserve respect. In chronic fatigue syndrome, what appears to be overprotection may arise from a belief that exertion makes things worse: which is true for that disease (it is also true that controlled exertion can make things better).

BOX 42.2 Case Example

> A 10-year-old boy with asthma is noted to have much poorer school attendance than the severity of his asthma, as judged by professionals, could justify. He often arrives in school late, and misses one or two days every week. Careful history taking elicits firstly that his mother tests his peak flow rate every morning, when it is often lower

than the rest of the day, and secondly that she had **two** relatives who died from status asthmaticus on the way into hospital. No-one can persuade her that his asthma will not become this severe, nor that her anxiety might be contributing to his tight chest in the morning. More flexible educational arrangements are necessary.

➤ *Social effects* – A chronic illness or lifelong handicap in a child may strain parents socially and financially as well as emotionally. If there are *two parents*, one may have to give up work, and the other may have to forgo promotion, in order to be available for the child. Financial difficulties may ensue. There may be little time for a social life, and other parents may be uncomprehending. Some relationships are strengthened by such duress, while others collapse. A *single parent* may find the strain inordinately difficult to cope with if unsupported: the difficulties others have in understanding the sorts of pressure involved can make her feel extremely isolated.

Effects on *siblings* include the following.
➤ *Feeling left out*. It is difficult for parents not to give the ill child more attention. Unaffected siblings may feel the ill child is more important, or that they have to be ill to get the same love and attention.

BOX 42.3 Case Example

The sister of a boy with acute myeloid leukaemia who has survived two bone marrow transplants – involving much travelling for their parents – develops severe abdominal pain, requiring admission to hospital. No organic cause is found.

➤ *Becoming parental* towards the ill or handicapped child. This seems to affect older siblings, particularly girls. This may have a beneficial effect on the sibling's development, providing she also has the chance to be an age-appropriate child.

Grandparents:
➤ **can be very helpful** as temporary childminders for the siblings and a support for parents
➤ may at times be **unhelpful** if they become critical of the parents' handling of the situation, or amplify their anxiety
➤ may experience a **double burden** of grief:
   — for their grandchild
   — for their child – a parent – who is so affected by the child's illness.

Other members of the extended family may find themselves in similar situations. Effects on *peers* may include the following.

➤ *Not understanding* what is going on, because no-one explains it. Teachers and other adults may not know, or if they do may feel understandably reluctant to breach confidentiality. A child's parents may be too distraught to consider the need of the child's friends for an appropriate explanation.

➤ *Misinformation* about the illness, for instance thinking that having to inject insulin means you are at risk of catching human immunodeficiency virus, or that having leukaemia means you are definitely going to die.

➤ Not having access to *support* in coping with their own feelings, such as worry about what may happen to their friend, or grief in response to the friend's death.

MANAGEMENT

As with CAMHS services in general, there is tremendous geographical variation in how services for the emotional health and wellbeing of children with chronic illness are provided. Some paediatric departments are lucky enough to have the support of a *paediatric liaison service* – which should consist of one or more child mental health professionals with specific responsibility for paediatric patients (both inpatient and outpatient) – but these are only patchily available.[3] Lesser degrees of support may be available from the specialist CAMHS team that provides outpatient services to the community, but unfortunately these teams do not always see the paediatric department as a priority. Whatever the level of specialist provision available, there is likely to be a role for primary care professionals, if only after hospital discharge. Local involvement may be centred in the community paediatric nursing service, but others with a more specific remit in mental health may contribute. Sometimes, the number of different professionals involved may require the appointment of a key worker or case coordinator, and regular multi-professional meetings involving everyone who is working with the child and family, to ensure that everyone works together without any gaps or unnecessary duplication.

The *support* needed by a child and family from primary care professionals will depend on the extent of the input from any specialist team involved. Resources to consider include support groups (for parents, affected children, or siblings); meeting other young people with similar conditions (particularly if the condition is too rare for there to be a local group); and charitable foundations for holidays. Support for the family needs to include practical considerations such as Disability Living Allowance and other benefits, arranging respite care if appropriate, and attending to the physical and emotional needs of all family members, especially siblings.

The child may need help to maintain *adherence* with recommended treatment, such as medication to be swallowed, insulin to be injected (in diabetes) or physiotherapy to be done (in cystic fibrosis). Education (just telling the young person what will happen if she doesn't do as she is told) is insufficient for this: behavioural methods are essential.[4]

Attention to *peers* may be an important aspect of holistic management. Classmates may need to be given basic information about the illness: this could be arranged between the class teacher and the community school nurse, community paediatric nurse, or specialist hospital nurse. Parents can be asked what specific information they will allow to be shared with the child's friends. If the child dies, close friends and probably many others in the same school – including teachers – may need some support. The head teacher may arrange to hold some sort of ritual or brief memorial in school assembly.

BOX 42.4 Case Example

Daphne has achondroplasia (a form of dwarfism). She copes very well in a small, supportive primary school. When she goes to a large secondary school at the age of 11, things become much more difficult for her. She starts calling herself a freak and becomes socially isolated. Despite being academically above average, Daphne's standard of schoolwork suffers. Her school Head of Year refers her to the school counsellor and primary mental health worker, who give her parents details of the nearest support group.[5] She finds it very useful to rehearse how she can explain to new acquaintances what makes her short. She also benefits greatly from a leg-lengthening operation. Gradually, she becomes more able to accept how different she is and slowly makes more friends.

BOX 42.5 Case Example

Shane, aged 13 years, suffers from Crohn's disease. He has recently moved schools and is noted to appear anxious at times. He is seen by the community school nurse, who elicits several worries he has about his illness. These include: the time he misses from school, keeping up with the work, using the school toilets, and having to leave the class quickly when needed. Shane describes being generally fed-up with the effect that the illness is having on him at present, and he is even beginning to wonder how it will affect his future life.

The community school nurse talks through these issues with Shane and then with his agreement discusses things with the primary mental health worker and his mother. The nurse then convenes a school meeting including herself, Shane, his parents, school staff and the primary mental health worker. The paediatrician cannot attend but discusses the situation with the community school nurse prior to the meeting.

It is agreed at the meeting that Shane will have access to the staff toilet near reception and will also be given a time-out card so he can leave lessons quickly if necessary. Shane is happy for all staff to be made aware of his medical condition. Shane's form tutor agrees to meet with Shane weekly to check his progress with work. If he is ill, worksheets and homework will be sent home via a friend – providing Shane feels well enough to work at home. Shane agrees to meet with the primary mental health worker fortnightly in the short-term to discuss some of his concerns about his illness. The community school nurse invites him to attend her drop-in clinic whenever he wishes. The group of professionals acknowledges to Shane that Crohn's disease is not an easy condition for anyone to cope with, and Shane appears to be managing remarkably well. They agreed to meet every term – as long as Shane finds this supportive.

Shane meets with the primary mental health worker for six sessions. He then reports feeling brighter in mood and more able to manage his illness and the impact it has on him. He says he does not need further appointments at present, but they agree he may in the future. He also continues to see his paediatrician regularly – who continues to liaise with the team around Shane, mainly via the community school nurse.

REFERRAL

Any referral to mental health services such as CAMHS or the primary mental health worker should ideally be from an involved paediatrician or someone who is part of the paediatric liaison services already working closely with the child.[5] This is so that any work with the family can be precisely coordinated. Many families find it difficult to accept the need for a referral to CAMHS services, preferring to keep the focus on paediatric problems. It may therefore be better to compile a local support package from other community primary care staff already involved, who can then, when necessary, consult for advice from CAMHS or the primary mental health worker.

BOX 42.6 Case Example

A child with a chronic illness and her family are just becoming comfortable with seeing the paediatric liaison psychologist, although initially they fear being told it is 'all in her mind'. Because of her difficulties at school, the special needs coordinator makes a referral to specialist CAMHS, without consulting the liaison psychologist or the consultant paediatrician first. The girl's parents take this as an implication that she must have a mental health problem. They do not attend the offered appointment at CAMHS and stop attending appointments with the liaison psychologist.

BOX 42.7 Practice Points for chronic illness

Psychological and social problems are more common in the presence of chronic physical illness.
Particular issues to think about include:
• the child's understanding of the illness
• the child's resilience
• the meaning attached by the family to the illness
• the effect of the illness on the child's family relationships
• the feelings of siblings
• parental coping strengths
• parental need for support from extended family and friends
• the financial impact of the illness

- the impact of the illness on peers
- the impact of the illness on teachers
- the possible need for respite.

RESOURCE: A BOOK FOR YOUNG PEOPLE

- Kaufman M. *Easy for You to Say: Q and A's for teens living with chronic illness or disability.* New York, NY: Firefly Books; 2005.
This is a straightforward and non-judgmental book of advice for teenagers with a wide range of illnesses.

REFERENCES

1 We are grateful for the input to this chapter from Dr Avril Washington, Consultant Paediatrician at Homerton University Hospital, London.

2 Pittet I, Berchtold A, Akré C, *et al.* Are adolescents with chronic conditions particularly at risk for bullying? *Arch Dis Child.* 2010; **95**(9): 711–16.

3 Kraemer S. Liaison and co-operation between paediatrics and mental health. *Paediatrics and Child Health.* 2010; **20**(8): 382–7.

4 Dean AJ, Walters J, Hall A. A systematic review of interventions to enhance medication adherence in children and adolescents with chronic illness. *Arch Dis Child.* 2010; **95**: 717–23.

5 www.achondroplasia.co.uk

PART 7

Specific issues

CHAPTER 43

Consent, competence, capacity and confidentiality

INTRODUCTION AND DEFINITIONS

All professionals working with children and their families have to be aware of and consider a range of issues relating to consent, competence, capacity and confidentiality. A plethora of guidance is available. This chapter aims to provide a brief summary of these issues and point to sources of information and advice.

Consent

Consent is the voluntary and continuing permission of a patient to receive a particular treatment, based on adequate knowledge of the purpose, nature, likely effects and risks of that treatment, including the likelihood of its success and any alternatives to it.

Informed consent requires:

➤ information
➤ capacity
➤ freedom to choose.

We will discuss capacity below, but first we need to look at the issue of parental responsibility.

Parental responsibility

Parental responsibility is defined in the Children Act 1989 as: 'All the rights, duties, powers, responsibilities and authority which by law a parent of a child has in relation to a child and his property'.[1] (The word 'child' in this Act refers to anyone under the age of 18.) Anyone under 18 is likely at times to need a parent to care for her, help her make a decision, or make a decision for her: this is both a privilege and an obligation. In practice, this may be done by anyone with a parental role, including step-parents or foster parents, and the Children Act states that a person who has care of a child without having parental responsibility for them may '... do what is reasonable in all the circumstances of the case for the purpose of safeguarding or promoting the child's welfare'. But legally, parental responsibility can be held by:

➤ the biological mother
➤ the biological father, if married to the mother at the time of birth or at some time thereafter

➤ the biological father, if the child was born after 1 December 2003 (England and Wales), 15 April 2002 (Northern Ireland) or 4 May 2006 (Scotland), and the father was registered on the child's birth certificate

➤ the biological father or stepfather, if he has applied to the court and been granted parental responsibility

➤ the mother's female civil partner, if she has agreed to the conception

➤ the adoptive parents, if the child has been adopted (in which case the biological parents lose parental responsibility)

➤ the child's social worker, if she is on a Care Order or Interim Care Order or Emergency Protection Order (in which case any biological parents with parental responsibility keep it, but their decisions can in principle be overridden by social services)

➤ anyone who has a Residence Order for the child

➤ anyone else who has applied successfully to the court for parental responsibility (this is most likely to be a relative in a parental role).

BOX 43.1 Case Example

When he is 10 years old, Robert's school refers him to the primary mental health worker because of concerns about his behaviour.

The primary mental health worker meets with Robert on his own and with his foster-mother. With the foster mother's permission, she discusses Robert with the school. She gathers the impression that Robert feels very different from others at his school as he has not grown up in the area, and as a black Caribbean, belongs to an ethnic minority that is uncommon locally. The primary mental health worker discovers rather belatedly that Robert is in a private fostering arrangement (not involving social services).

Robert wants to spend more time with his natural mother, who lives about fifty miles away. The primary mental health worker tries to contact Robert's mother by writing to her. The response is a complaint from mother that Robert has been taken to see a mental health professional without her consent, and that the school has become too involved in private family matters.

The primary mental health worker seeks advice from her manager and the local social services legal department. It emerges that the foster mother has a letter signed by the mother enabling her to obtain any necessary healthcare. Robert's mother states that she meant this to apply only to physical health. Like most foster carers, the foster mother does not have parental responsibility, but unlike most foster carers, she has never been approved by social services.

The primary mental health worker's manager meets with Robert's natural mother and explains that the primary mental health worker was acting in good faith but should in retrospect have ensured she had adequate parental consent before contacting the school (and the school should ideally have sought parental consent before making the referral, but was used to working with the foster mother). Robert's mother does not pursue her complaint.

Legally, it is sufficient to have the consent of one person with parental responsibility for any mental health intervention. However, it is often prudent to enquire about others with parental responsibility, and consider asking for their views. This is likely to be a particular problem when parents have separated, but both retain a parenting role.

BOX 43.2 Case Example

Timothy, aged eight years, is brought to his local community paediatric ADHD clinic by his mother with a request for an ADHD assessment. The outcome of this is a diagnosis of ADHD. Timothy's mother says she would like a trial of medication. The consultant paediatrician prescribes methylphenidate.

Two weeks later, the community paediatrician receives a letter from Timothy's father saying that he does not agree with this plan. The parents separated acrimoniously when Timothy was three years old, but he has fortnightly staying contact with his father.

The community paediatrician agrees to meet with Timothy's father. It emerges that he was married to Timothy's mother when Timothy was born, so he has parental responsibility. He isn't convinced by the diagnosis of ADHD, saying that Timothy is fine with him, and he is very opposed to the use of medication.

The community paediatrician seeks advice from his trust's solicitors. They suggest either mediation or an appeal to the courts. The parents both say they do not want to sit in the same room with any mediator (not even the community paediatrician), and mother says she does not want to go to court about this issue, so father's veto on medication is allowed to stand.

The Zone of Parental Control

This concept derives from the Mental Health Act 2007 and case law in the European Court of Human Rights in Strasbourg.[2] It means what an adult can decide about a child under 16 or a young person of 16 or 17 for whom she has parental responsibility. Medical procedures on children under 16 would normally fall within the Zone of Parental Control, providing:

➤ The decision is one that a parent would normally be expected to make. More extreme interventions are likely to fall outside the zone.

➤ There are no indications that the parent might not act in the best interests of the child. If there could be a conflict of interest for the parent (as might occur after an acrimonious divorce), or if the child has alleged abuse by the parent, then professionals may decide to restrict the Zone of Parental Control.

➤ There is no reason to suppose the parent lacks the capacity to consent (for instance due to substance misuse or learning disability).

➤ The young person agrees with the treatment proposed. If the young person is resisting, then more justification is needed to use parental consent alone.

Decisions regarding 16 and 17 year olds are likely to fall within the Zone of Parental Control only if the young person lacks the ability to consent for himself.

BOX 43.3 Case Example

> Alice is a 13-year-old girl whose mother takes her to Accident and Emergency with acute abdominal pain. Surgical assessment suggests probable appendicitis requiring exploratory surgery. There are signs of inflammation, but the appendix does not seem to have burst yet. Alice says she does not want an operation, because she is terrified. The casualty officer suggests a mental health assessment. The consultant surgeon states this is quite unnecessary, as the decision is within the zone of parental control, and he is prepared to operate with mother's consent only. The operation goes ahead, and Alice feels much better afterwards.

BOX 43.4 Case Example

> Pauline is a 13-year-old girl who is taken to Accident and Emergency by her grandmother, with whom she is staying temporarily. She has signs of a perforated appendix, a high fever, is confused, and will not agree to anything. The surgical registrar states that she needs emergency surgery. Pauline's grandmother cannot contact either of her parents, who are on holiday abroad in an area without mobile phone reception. The surgical registrar asks grandmother to sign the consent form. The casualty officer, who has been reading too many books, points out that this consent is not legally valid. The registrar telephones his consultant, who points out that consent is not necessary for emergency procedures, which can be done under common law if they are required to save life or prevent severe deterioration. The operation goes ahead, and Pauline's parents write the Registrar a thank you letter after their return from holiday.

Gillick competence and Fraser guidelines

This relates to whether the young person understands the nature of the decision and has sufficient maturity to deal with the consequences. It arose as a result of a legal case following the prescription of contraceptives to an under-16 year old without her mother's consent.

The term 'Gillick competence' is sometimes replaced by the term 'Fraser guidelines' (named after the judge rather than the mother of the young person whose case these are based on). These should be considered not only when making a decision about prescribing contraceptives under 16, but also in a range of other contexts. To be Gillick competent to receive a contraceptive prescription without parental knowledge or consent, a young person:

➤ should understand relevant professional advice and its implications
➤ cannot be persuaded to inform her parents

➤ is likely to begin, or to continue having, sexual intercourse with or without contraceptive treatment
➤ is likely to suffer, with regard to her physical or mental health, unless she receives contraceptive treatment
➤ the young person's best interests require her to receive contraceptive advice or treatment with or without parental consent.

These principles can be generalised to any situation in which a young person's consent may be valid without involvement of a person with parental responsibility: ranging from any medical, surgical or dental treatment to issues such as parental contact. The young person must have 'sufficient age and understanding' in relation to the issue in question: Gillick competence is specific to one issue, and can vary for different issues. For instance, an 11 year old may be Gillick competent to decide whether she should see her absent father, but a 15 year old may not be competent to give or withhold consent for a heart transplant.

THE ASSESSMENT OF COMPETENCE IN YOUNG PEOPLE

Competence may be influenced by:
➤ emotional development
➤ intellectual capacity
➤ mental illness such as psychosis or depression
➤ pressures from peers, parents or media
➤ personality (for instance: excessive stubbornness, flip-flop decision-making, a tendency to agree with what the last person has said, or being mature and balanced in approach to decisions)
➤ the young person's relationship with relevant professionals.

When assessing a young person's competence, the clinician needs to consider:
➤ stage of development
➤ the parent-child relationship
➤ the doctor-patient relationship
➤ the views of significant others
➤ the risks and benefits of treatment
➤ the nature of the illness
➤ the need for consensus.[3]

BOX 43.5 Case Example

Esmeralda, a 15-year-old girl, is brought to Accident and Emergency by her mother two hours after an overdose of 32 paracetomol tablets. After an hour's wait, she announces that she is going home, and her mother calls a nurse. The nurse in charge phones the Accident and Emergency Consultant on call to express her concern about letting Esmeralda go. His view is that:
• Esmeralda can be kept in under common law until a psychiatric assessment can be done

> • She is probably not (Gillick) competent to decide what is best for her if she has felt bad enough to take such a large overdose, so keeping her in against her will falls within the Zone of Parental Control. In the short term, it can therefore be left up to her mother to decide whether Esmeralda should be kept in hospital forcibly.

Capacity

Capacity has the following components. The patient:
➤ has the ability to comprehend and retain treatment information
➤ is able to weigh the information in balance
➤ is able to arrive at a free choice
➤ has the ability to communicate this.

With young people, information has to be tailored to their needs, whilst recognising that their ability to come to a free choice may be compromised. Health professionals must assess the capacity to consent for a particular treatment proposal at the time the treatment is proposed. The Family Law Reform Act 1969 makes the presumption of capacity for young people aged 16 plus. For under-16s, the onus is on the clinician to demonstrate that the young person has capacity and – for those over 16 – to show he or she does *not* have capacity.

The Mental Capacity Act (2005) provides a legal framework for decision making on behalf of anyone aged 16 or over who lacks the capacity to make specific decisions for himself.[4] Capacity is specific to a particular decision and a particular time, for instance whether to have an indicated treatment or not. It is defined by the Act in a negative way, as follows.

A person over 16 can be considered unable to make a particular decision only if:
1 He or she has 'an impairment of, or disturbance in the functioning of the mind or brain', whether permanent or temporary; *AND*
2 He or she is unable to undertake any of the following steps:
   ➤ understand the information relevant to the decision
   ➤ retain that information for long enough to come to a decision
   ➤ use or weigh that information as part of the process of making the decision
   ➤ communicate the decision made (whether by talking, sign language or other means).

Impaired capacity in 16 and 17 year olds may for instance be due to: high fever, severe learning difficulties, a psychotic episode, life-threatening self-harm, or severe restrictive anorexia nervosa. The Mental Capacity Act can be used to justify a particular procedure or treatment only if it does not entail deprivation of liberty.

Clinical problems do not always have straightforward solutions, and it is important whenever there is any doubt to discuss your options with clinical colleagues and others, including for instance: your professional body, any source of reliable legal advice, or your local Clinical Ethics Committee, if you have access to one.[5]

BOX 43.6 Case Example

Peter, aged 16, is at a special school for children with severe learning difficulties; he communicates mainly by sign language. One day, while at home, he swallows some bleach. It is not clear whether he meant to harm himself, but he has been throwing things at his parents more than usual recently, and he has been upset by the death of the family golden retriever. Assessment in Accident and Emergency indicates that he needs to stay in hospital for monitoring, intravenous fluids and endoscopy, but Peter is unhappy with the strange environment, and indicates that he very much wants to go home. As the proposed treatment involves deprivation of liberty, the Mental Capacity Act cannot be used. After discussion with Peter's parents, involved professionals agree that the proposed management is within the Zone of Parental Control. Peter is kept in hospital, and his parents consent to the necessary investigations and treatment on his behalf.

BOX 43.7 Case Example

Paul is a 15-year-old boy living in a children's home. He presents to Accident and Emergency following a reaction to Ecstasy. He is reluctant to say how much he has taken, but he has clear psychotic symptoms including seeing ants crawling all over the walls. He is more scared of these than the hospital and can be persuaded relatively easily to stay on the children's ward, although he needs to be in a cubicle close to the nursing station so he can be closely observed. It emerges that the only person with parental responsibility is his mother, who has infrequent contact with Paul. She is abroad, and no one – including Paul – knows a contact number for her. The professional consensus is that Paul lacks capacity and Gillick competence to consent to treatment but can be treated under common law. The Mental Capacity Act does not apply because he is under 16. His recovery is hastened by the use of olanzapine, which he agrees to take when it is explained to him that it will make the ants go away.

BOX 43.8 Case Example

Erica is 17 years old and has had restrictive anorexia nervosa for two years. She is currently vomiting after every meal, intensively exercising, and losing weight at the rate of at least 0.5 kg per week. She is found to have a low potassium of 2.5 but refuses to come into hospital, saying she hates the place. There is no psychiatric bed immediately available within easy visiting distance for her parents. Recommended treatment involves intravenous fluids with potassium, nasogastric feeding, and close monitoring, particularly of her phosphate. Although she lacks capacity, the Mental Capacity Act cannot be used as she is not agreeing to admission. There is some doubt as to whether the proposed management falls within the Zone of Parental Control, and nurses are concerned about what they would do if Erica tried to leave the ward. After discussion between parents, paediatricians, paediatric nurses and child mental health professionals, it is agreed that the most appropriate way forward is the Mental Health Act 1983/2007. Erica is admitted to the paediatric ward on Section 3 for two weeks, with round-the-clock psychiatric nursing, until a local psychiatric bed becomes available. While on the paediatric ward, she has to accept the necessary nutritional treatment, since it is for her psychiatric condition.

BOX 43.9 Continuation of Case Example in Box 43.6

Peter gets home after his hospital admission, but his behaviour continues to be challenging for his parents. They very much do not want him to go into a residential home if they can avoid it. He refuses to take tablets or liquid. Eventually it is agreed that his parents will conceal risperidone liquaid in his meals, but Peter's parents and the prescribing doctor feel unhappy about doing this on a long-term basis, so the Mental Capacity Act is used to justify treatment.

INFORMATION SHARING

The tragic case of Victoria Climbié, a once happy, smiling, enthusiastic little girl brought to England by a relative for 'a better life' who died following severe, cruel abuse led to an inquiry chaired by Lord Laming. In his report he concluded that: 'The extent of the failure to protect Victoria was lamentable' and that 'The suffering and death of Victoria was a gross failure of the system and was inexcusable'.[6] Lord Laming made a number of recommendations to address the failures in the system that had contributed to her death, many of which have been embodied in the collection of executive and organisational changes referred to as 'Every Child Matters'.[7]

What happened to Victoria led to those working with and having contact with children to reconsider the issue of information sharing between professionals and agencies, especially where there are concerns about the young person's well-being and/or the possibility of some form of child abuse (*see also* Chapter 12 on Child Abuse and Safeguarding).

When, why and how?

All people working with children/young people and their families need to think about when, why and how information should be shared in their daily practice. Information sharing is essential to enable children and families to receive the help and support they need as well as to safeguard and promote the welfare of children and young people. Key factors in many serious case reviews have been failures in areas such as:

➤ recording significant information
➤ sharing it with other professionals who can appreciate its significance and do something about it

➤ understanding the significance of the information shared
➤ taking appropriate action in relation to known or suspected abuse or neglect.

Confidential information

This refers to sensitive information that is shared with another person when the person giving the information understood it would not be shared with others. Confidence is breached only when this information is passed onto someone else without the young person's authorisation. Seeking consent to share information should be routine; however, there may be circumstances when it is appropriate (and lawful) to pass on information even without the young person's consent, for instance if there is a clear risk of significant harm to any child.

Safeguarding and confidentiality

The general rule is that child protection (now more often called 'safeguarding') trumps confidentiality. If there is a risk of significant harm happening to any child or young person, or continuing to happen, if the information is not passed on, then it is justifiable to break a young person's confidence. It is, however, good practice to inform the young person before doing this, as this will probably maintain the young person's trust. If you say, for instance: 'What you have told me is very serious, and I probably need to pass it on to other professionals' or 'I am not sure whether I need to inform the police and social services about this, but I will ask a colleague, and I may have to do it even though you may not want me to. Do you understand why?' – then most young people will understand the kind of duty you are explaining to them – although they may be discouraged from telling you any more.

Judgement needs to be exercised over whether to tell a parent or not: the general rule is that it is usually courteous and therefore best practice to warn parents what you are likely to do unless this either:
➤ puts a child at more risk; or
➤ jeopardises a likely police investigation.

It is advisable to check your local safeguarding guidelines, or ask your local safeguarding nurse or doctor.

BOX 43.10 Case Example

Gemma, aged 14 years, is seeing the primary mental health worker for weekly individual sessions with regard to her low mood. In one of her sessions she discloses that her father has been physically chastising her younger brothers. Whilst he is not hurting her because she keeps out of his way when he is angry, Gemma is worried about her brothers and their well-being – but she does not want her father to know that she has said anything. Initially, she is very anxious about this information being shared with anyone, but after further discussion, she agrees that this information can initially be shared with her mother.

Gemma's mother admits that there are difficulties at home and that she too has seen the physical chastisement of the children – she has felt unsure what to do about it. The primary mental health worker explains that, in light of this information, she needs to make a referral to social services. Gemma is relieved that her mother is now also aware of the situation and that she knows about social services having to be informed, although both Gemma and her mother are worried that social services might remove her younger brothers from the family home.

A duty social worker visits the family. Gemma's father admits he has been losing it with the children more than usual recently and starts crying. The social worker thinks he appears depressed, and persuades him to visit the general practitioner with his wife. The general practitioner also thinks Gemma's father is suffering from depression. Gemma's father agrees to see the practice counsellor and take antidepressants.

Gemma continues to see the primary mental health worker weekly. She reports a gradual improvement in the situation at home. After a couple of months, she no longer feels any concern for the safety of her younger brothers. She also starts to feel happier and more confident in herself and is able to reduce and then stop her sessions with the primary mental health worker.

BOX 43.11 Case Example

One of the pupils at a secondary school passes a note to a teacher written by another pupil, Jack, aged 15 years. In this note, Jack describes how low he feels and mentions the possibility of hanging himself in the barn of a farm near where he lives.

The teacher approaches Jack, who becomes very upset and states he has no intention of killing himself. He insists that he does not want his parents to know about the note, in case they become angry or upset.

The teacher explains that she cannot possibly keep this information secret, however much Jack wants her to. This is the sort of information she simply has to pass on to his parents – because they are his parents, and they need to know if there is any possibility that he might kill himself.

She gets hold of Jack's parents as soon as she can by telephone. They collect Jack from school and take him to his general practitioner for an urgent appointment. This leads in turn to an urgent appointment in specialist CAMHS.

BOX 43.12 Case Example

Sarah, aged 15 years, visits the Community School Nurse in her drop-in clinic. She starts to discuss her anxiety about impending exams and the impact of her parents' recent bitter divorce. She does not want her parents to be informed of her contact.

The community school nurse agrees with Sarah that their meetings can remain confidential, but with the proviso that she will have to inform Sarah's parents if she ever feels Sarah (or anyone else) is at risk of harm. Sarah appears to accept this.

Sarah visits the community school nurse regularly over the next two terms. Gradually, she agrees to let the community school nurse share with her form tutor some of the difficulty she is having organising her GCSE coursework, and he is able to suggest some study skills and ways of pacing the work, as well as renegotiate some deadlines. Sarah seems relieved to be able to share with him her feelings about the war between her parents.

Sarah's parents are not informed of what she is going through. Her anxiety symptoms improve.

BOX 43.13 Case Example

Hannah is 14 years old and gets on well with her personal and social education teacher. One day, Hannah asks to see her at the end of a lesson. To the teacher's surprise, Hannah discloses that she is worried that her younger sister, aged 12, is going to be sexually abused by their father. The teacher is not sure how to respond but asks Hannah what makes her think this. Hannah says she would rather not explain. The teacher says she will need to take advice about what to do with this information. The teacher again asks if there is anything else that Hannah would like to say. Hannah says no and rushes home.

The next day, the teacher manages to persuade Hannah to talk to her in a private place. She explains that she has talked to the school's safeguarding adviser (a deputy head teacher), who has suggested that if Hannah has good reasons for suspecting that her father will abuse her sister, she will need to explain them to social services. The fact that she has told a teacher something suggests that she would like to protect her sister. Hannah nods her head to both of these statements. The teacher then asks Hannah if she would be prepared to say more to social services than she has been able to say to her. Hannah says she is not sure, but she thinks she would prefer to talk to someone she knows. The teacher explains that she will have to make a referral to social services whether Hannah likes it or not, and Hannah looks very scared. The teacher asks her why she looks scared, and Hannah says she cannot say. She asks the teacher not to tell her mother, to which the teacher reluctantly agrees.

When the social worker visits Hannah in school, Hannah will not give any more reasons for her concern. She refuses the suggestion of a videotaped interview with the police. By the time the social worker interviews Hannah's mother at her workplace, Hannah has told her mother that the teacher misunderstood her and has blown everything out of proportion. The social worker obtains mother's consent to interview Hannah's younger sister, who says she has nothing to fear from their father. At the subsequent professionals' meeting, which does not include Hannah or her parents, the teachers and social workers agree that there are grounds for grave concern, but that they can do nothing further unless Hannah is prepared to explain her fears in more detail.

GMC guidance for doctors

The General Medical Council, which regulates doctors and encourages good medical practice, has produced a helpful body of guidance for doctors that can also be useful for other professionals working with children and young people.[8] This covers the following areas:

➤ assessing best interests
➤ effective communication
➤ making decisions and the capacity to consent
➤ principles of confidentiality and information sharing
➤ access to medical records by children, young people and their parents
➤ sexual activity
➤ contraception, abortions and sexually transmitted infections
➤ suitability to work with children and young people
➤ prescribing medicines
➤ other sources of information and guidance, legislation and case law and useful links.

BOX 43.14 Case Example

Jennifer, aged 12 years, has been seeing the community school nurse about her unhappiness. She blames this partly on being ostracised at school and partly on her parents' divorce when she was nine years old. The school nurse has obtained Jennifer's mother's consent to see Jennifer, and has obtained Jennifer's consent to see her mother. She has held two joint appointments to get some background information about the family but has not met Jennifer's father, whom Jennifer visits every other weekend. The other eight appointments have been with Jennifer alone.

Out of the blue, the nurse receives a letter from Jennifer's father asking to see the nurse's notes, stating he believes his ex-wife has provided biased information. The nurse takes advice from her trust customer services department. They suggest that the nurse should try to be as obliging as possible, but should ascertain Jennifer's and her mother's views first. She informs Jennifer of her father's letter. Jennifer is rather upset, describing her father as controlling and having dominated her mother in the last years of their marriage, which fits with mother's description. Jennifer does not want her father to see her notes, and does not want the nurse to offer father a meeting. Jennifer's mother says she is willing to support Jennifer's wishes and does not want to have a joint meeting with father. She has no particular wish to see Jennifer's notes herself.

The nurse composes a joint letter to Jennifer's father with her manager, which they show to the trust's customer services department before sending. In it, the nurse writes that she agrees that the information she has been given is bound to be biased, as it is from only one party in the divorce. However, her first duty is to her patient, Jennifer, and Jennifer will not give her consent for her father to see her notes. She states that she has taken advice from colleagues and has decided that

Jennifer is competent to make a decision on this issue. Jennifer subsequently reports that her father has put pressure on her to change her mind, but she has instead refused to visit him for three consecutive fortnights. Eventually she returns, and her father does not bring up the issue again.

Practical considerations

Some key points on information sharing are summarised here.

➤ Explain to the young person and his family at the outset why, what, when and how information will be shared and seek their agreement (unless this would put them or others at risk of significant harm or interfere with the investigation of a serious crime).

➤ Consider the child's welfare and safety when making decisions about whether to share information about them.

➤ Respect the young person's wishes (where possible).

➤ If in doubt, seek advice from a colleague or your manager/supervisor.

➤ Ensure any information shared is accurate, up to date and needs to be shared.

➤ Record the reasons for your decision.

Employers/agencies should have clear advice and policies about this that dovetail with local safeguarding procedures.

In practice, when a parent/carer brings a child to see you, the child's consent to the interview may be assumed. The child's understanding of what is happening should be established by explaining who you are, why you are meeting and what you are going to do (and *not* do – young children may associate a health professional with a previous unpleasant experience, such as a blood test or injection).

Begin by explaining your role and involvement; for instance: 'I am [name and simplified job description]. I see children who . . . Do you know X? He asked me to see you. He was worried about . . .' Then explain what is going to happen; for instance: 'I'd like to begin by talking with both of you, and then I would like to spend some time with you on your own.' Acknowledge there may be things to talk about that are sensitive or confidential and be prepared to be flexible: 'Sometimes, there are things parents or young people would rather say on their own . . . that's all right . . . we can make a separate appointment to do that . . . or see you each on your own if that would be better . . .' A clear statement about confidentiality can be made at the outset, before any issues arise. Do not promise confidentiality if asked to by the young person, but clarify when you may have to share information (*see* Alarm Bells in Box 43.15).

If your agency/service has written forms about information sharing and consent, consider when and how to present these. Sometimes, basic information gathering and information about the service is sent to the family before an appointment. At other times, using the forms during the session may be best but beware of the danger of form-filling taking over and hindering the process of getting to know the young person, building a trusting relationship with her and finding out what is really going on.

Do not agree to hear information in total confidence. If the conversation starts with: 'I want to tell you a secret' or 'You must promise not to tell …' you must clarify with the individual that you cannot guarantee that what she says will be kept private if someone is at risk of harm.

BOX 43.15 Alarm Bells in the management of confidentiality

Things a young person may say:
'Will you promise to keep a secret?'
'I am not telling you anything unless you promise not to tell anyone.'
'I am scared of telling anyone anything more.'
Things a carer may say:
A parent may be very reluctant for you to spend part of the assessment alone with the child.
A parent may demand to see the notes you have kept on her child.
Something another professional may say:
A teacher or other professional could ask for details of what a child may have told you in confidence (when there are no concerns about safeguarding).

SUMMARY

Consent, capacity and confidentiality can be complex issues, particularly during the few years before and after a young person's 16th birthday. Most of the work done by professionals at Tier 1 and Tier 2 will be with the tacit consent of child or parent or both, but it may at times be important to consider:

➤ who holds parental responsibility?
➤ are the decisions requiring consent within the Zone of Parental Control?
➤ is the young person Gillick competent in relation to issues requiring her consent?
➤ does the young person have the capacity required to make relevant decisions?
➤ does the parent have the capacity required to make relevant decisions?
➤ is there a reason to break confidentiality?
➤ whom would it be advisable to ask before doing this?

REFERENCES

1 Her Majesty's Government. The Children Act 1989. London: Her Majesty's Stationery Office; 1989.
2 Department of Health. Code of Practice: Mental Health Act 1983 (revised for Mental Health Act 2007). London: The Stationery Office; 2008.
3 Pearce J. Consent to treatment during childhood: the assessment of competence and avoidance of conflict. British Journal of Psychiatry. 1994; 165(6): 713–16.

4 British Psychological Society, Royal College of Psychiatrists and Department of Health. Mental Capacity Act 2005: short reference guide for psychologists and psychiatrists, 2007. Available at: www.bps.org.uk (accessed 5 April 2011).

5 www.ethics-network.org.uk

6 The Victoria Climbié Inquiry: report of an inquiry by Lord Laming: www.dh.gov.uk/en/ Publicationsandstatistics/Publications/PublicationsPolicyAndGuidance/DH_4008654

7 www.dcsf.gov.uk/everychildmatters

8 General Medical Council. Zero to 18 years: guidance for doctors. London: General Medical Council; 2007. Available at: www.gmc-uk.org/guidance (accessed 5 April 2011).

CHAPTER 44

Diet and exercise

INTRODUCTION

Diet can make an important contribution to physical and mental health at any age.[1,2] There is emerging evidence that a child's diet may have a positive or negative influence on concentration, behaviour and achievement.[3] The importance of exercise cannot be overestimated, and all health professionals should take every opportunity to encourage it. The two are obviously connected, but we will discuss each in turn.

Diet

Aspects of *diet* that may have relevance to child mental health include the following.

➤ The omega-3 *highly unsaturated fatty acids* docosahexaenoic acid (DHA) and eicosapentaenoic acid (EPA) are relatively deficient in most Western diets, compared to: the 'Mediterranean' diet. DHA and EPA are important for the structure and optimal function of nerve cells in the brain and spinal cord. There is no generally recognised specific clinical syndrome associated with deficiency of these, but a relative deficiency may be a contributing factor in dyslexia, dyspraxia, ADHD, autistic spectrum disorder, antisocial behaviour, self-harm and depression.

  — In an extraordinary longitudinal study, the amount of maternal fish intake during pregnancy was found to predict the child's fine motor and social development at age 42 months, and the child's *prosocial abilities* and *verbal intelligence quotient* at age eight years.[4]

  — An intervention study in young people with *early signs of psychosis* showed much reduced progression to full psychosis after omega-3 supplementation.[5]

  — A pilot study of omega-3 supplementation in *childhood depression* had promising results.[6]

  — Although unselected children with ADHD seem not to respond significantly to omega-3 supplementation,[7] some *ADHD symptoms* do seem to respond,[8,9] including attention deficit[10] and working memory.[11]

  — *Reading and spelling* have also been found to improve with omega-3 supplementation.[12]

➤ Food *colourings* such as tartrazine or *preservatives* such as benzoate may cause any child to become more hyperactive and difficult to manage.[13,14]

➤ *Salt intake* – Salt is necessary to enable the body to function, but a consistent excess in childhood may contribute to population trends in adulthood towards high blood pressure.

➤ A diet with a high content of **refined carbohydrate** (such as sugar or white bread) may lead to surges of blood glucose and insulin that are less conducive to sustained mental or physical effort than the continuing absorption from the gut provided by unrefined complex carbohydrates, as found in most fruits, vegetables and whole grains. This is expressed as a number by the 'glycaemic index', which is 100 for glucose, and approaches this for white bread, white rice, baked potatoes and some cereals (such as Corn Flakes and Rice Krispies). This was originally developed as an aid for diabetics in managing their diet to minimise fluctuations in blood sugar, but has since been found to help those without diabetes. Eating a diet with low or medium glycaemic index can help to prevent obesity, heart disease and maturity-onset diabetes. The evidence for a direct impact on child mental health seems however to be limited.

➤ A **low fibre** diet (without sufficient unrefined carbohydrate, fruits or vegetables) may also predispose to constipation, which may have an impact on mood, either directly, or because of the emotional consequences of faecal incontinence (*see* Chapter 24: Faecal Incontinence).

➤ **Vitamin** deficiencies are rare in affluent countries because of supplementation put in a variety of foodstuffs, such as breakfast cereals or margarine. It is still possible for children to be deficient in some vitamins; for instance, rickets still occurs in the UK due to vitamin D deficiency, and scurvy can occur in children who eat little fruit, fruit juice or potatoes.

➤ A deficiency of **iron**, which is very common in the general population – particularly in infants and menstruating girls – may cause non-specific symptoms such as fatigue, malaise or poor concentration.

➤ Some **minerals**, such as zinc or magnesium, and **trace elements**, such as chromium and manganese, which are essential to the diet but only in small quantities, may cause a reduction in general well-being if deficient. ADHD has been linked to iodine deficiency via its effects on maternal thyroid function during pregnancy in a particular region of Italy.[15] Zinc supplementation has been suggested for ADHD.[16]

➤ **Multiple supplementation** of the diet with a mixture of vitamins, minerals and omega-3 fatty acids in incarcerated young offenders decreased antisocial behaviour,[17] an effect that has been replicated in Holland.[18]

➤ An imbalance between calorie input (how much you absorb from what you eat) and calorie output (basal metabolic rate plus calories used for exercise plus calories used to create body heat) can lead to **obesity**, which is reaching endemic proportions in affluent countries. This in turn can have an adverse impact not only on physical but also on mental health, the latter including for instance:
— low self-esteem
— becoming a victim of weight-related teasing or bullying
— comfort eating (creating a vicious circle)
— preoccupation with food
— eating disorders such as bulimia nervosa or binge-eating disorder.

Putting all this together could lead to dietary restriction and/or the use of supplement pills, but both entail their own risks. An emphasis on dieting (meaning restricting calories) can paradoxically lead to becoming overweight or to eating disorders such as anorexia nervosa or bulimia.[19] Using dietary supplements of vitamins, minerals or essential fatty acids, unless done carefully, could entail the risk of having too much of some things, which may create its own problems.

The healthiest path is likely to consist of eating a mixed diet with appropriate amounts of different food groups. Fruit, vegetables and nuts, for instance, can provide vitamins, minerals, trace elements and fibre, as well as some gradually absorbed carbohydrates, in roughly the right proportions. For an example of a balanced diet, *see*:

www.food.gov.uk/multimedia/pdfs/publication/eatwellplate0907.pdf

The difficulty with implementing the sort of healthy balanced diet shown in this diagram is that many children in the Western world do not eat like this. They are more likely to eat as shown in Figure 44.1, which is based on 24-hour recall diaries kept by Scottish primary school children, most of whom were between nine and 11 years of age.[20]

A child's eating habits may be influenced by some or all of the following factors:
➤ the child's temperament – for instance:
— is he more likely to go for short-term satisfaction or longer-term well-being?
— is he an exploratory child who enjoys trying new foods or an obsessional child who prefers to maintain sameness?
— is he likely to do what he is told or the opposite of what he is told?
➤ peer pressure
➤ parental modelling and family food culture
➤ use of certain foods as rewards by parents or others (for instance, using sweets as rewards will make them desirable; using apples or raisins as rewards will make *them* desirable)
➤ the success or otherwise of parents' efforts to get him to eat a healthy diet
➤ school's food policy
➤ what he chooses to have or eat in his packed lunches or school dinners

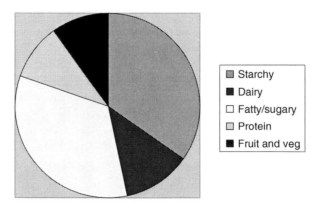

FIGURE 44.1 Proportions of foods actually eaten by children

➤ the shops he passes or is likely to use to buy snacks
➤ advertising
➤ financial factors, such as how much if anything his parents give him to spend on food of his choice.[21]

Not only do dietary imbalances potentially lead to child mental health problems, but family mental health issues may influence the child's diet.

BOX 44.1 Case Example

> Judy seeks advice from her health visitor about her four-year-old daughter Lucy's eating. Although there are no concerns about Lucy's weight, her diet consists mainly of bread products, bananas, yoghurt and plain pasta. Whenever Lucy is offered anything different, either at home or playschool, she will refuse with an adamant 'yuk'. Judy is increasingly anxious about this, as Lucy is due to start school soon, and she is worried that Lucy may become distressed at school mealtimes.
>
> Assessment reveals that Judy was also a fussy eater as a child and preferred to eat the same small range of foods each day. She describes her own childhood as limited in terms of the range of foods she was offered. This may be partly why she is unsure about what foods she should now be giving Lucy and how best to respond to Lucy's food refusal.
>
> The health visitor begins by discussing the range of food groups that make up a healthy diet using the Eatwell Plate – see www.food.gov.uk/multimedia/pdfs/publi cation/eatwellplate0907.pdf – and some fun ways of encouraging Lucy to try new foods. These activities include: games that involve tasting new foods, helping to pre-pare food, and presenting food in a child-friendly way using child-appropriate portion sizes. The health visitor also suggests that Judy could borrow from the local library some cookery books aimed to support healthy eating in young children.
>
> Judy finds that with a little gentle persuasion Lucy eventually tries different foods. Lucy gradually increases the variety in her diet.

Exercise

Regular participation in physical games and a variety of activities can not only help the development of fine and gross motor skills, but also help to prevent obesity. Factors making it difficult for children to take enough exercise include the following.
➤ The National Curriculum in UK schools does not build in sufficient regular exercise – due partly to other timetabling demands.
➤ Walking or cycling to school tends to be perceived by many parents as unsafe. While fears of 'stranger danger' may be statistically unfounded, these tend to be exaggerated by the media. The danger of traffic for children who walk or cycle is very real.

➤ There is pressure on land that in the past might have been available as a communal play space. Those playgrounds that remain are generally very safe and attractive to younger children, but many children have fewer opportunities than they would like for football, skateboarding or other group run-arounds.

➤ The effects of technology have encouraged sedentary activities by the whole family. Many households may be dominated by screen-centred activities, such as television, DVDs, console games or personal computers. It can be very tempting for parents to allow the technology to do some 'babysitting' and have some time to themselves, rather than struggling to impose limits on the amount of time each child spends spellbound by a screen.

➤ Many parents find it difficult to set an example to their children of integrating exercise into everyday life. Sedentary jobs and travel to work inside vehicles is too often combined with sedentary leisure activities.

Assessment

An assessment of the child's dietary input and exercise can be made informally by going through the child's regular day, perhaps differentiating school days from non-school days, enquiring about what he eats for each meal and snack, and the nature of activities. A more formal assessment may involve providing structured dairies and advice about how to record periods of exercise and food eaten – which may require input from a paediatric dietician.

MANAGEMENT AND REFERRAL

Diet

The dietary habits of many children leave room for improvement, as shown at www.food.gov.uk/multimedia/pdfs/publication/eatwellplate0907.pdf, and are potentially an important contributor to psychological health and mental well-being. How can we improve dietary habits?

➤ *Parents* can be advised to help the child develop a healthy eating pattern in a variety of ways.
  — Encourage the child to explore new tastes and textures from an early age.
  — Make healthy foods exciting, by using them as rewards or special treats – for example, apples or raisins.
  — Make sure there are plenty of healthy foods available in the household to snack on, such as fresh fruits, dried fruits (and nuts as long as there are no allergies or children young enough to choke on them).
  — Limit the availability of foods high in fat, sugar, salt, colourings and preservatives.
  — Limit the whole family's access to fast food.
  — Provide plentiful fibre, for instance in brown bread, vegetables and fruits.
  — Model the way you want your child to eat by eating that way yourself: many children will want to eat what they see a parent eating.
➤ *Schools* can be assisted in making available food more nutritious *and* enjoyable.[22]
  — They can ensure that meals and snacks available to all pupils make a contribution to a healthy diet.

- School canteens can influence buying preferences by the way that food is arranged.[23]
➤ *Government*, probably more central than local, can legislate in the following ways.
  - *Food producers* can be guided to make their foods healthier, for instance by regulating the amount of added iron in bread or breakfast cereals (as is already done) or reducing unsaturated fat or sugar in foods.
  - *Advertisers* can be prevented from targeting advertisements at children that make them want more unhealthy food.
  - *Shops* where children buy snacks and other foods could be given profit-related incentives to sell more healthy food and less unhealthy food.
  - A programme of *differential taxation* could make it easier for parents to afford healthy food rather than unhealthy food.

Other aspects of dietary behaviour may involve child mental health professionals. Some parents use *exclusion diets* to treat a child, for instance if the child has autistic spectrum disorder or ADHD. Many parents note a child becoming more hyperactive on certain foods: research has confirmed that this is a valid observation.[24] At the time of writing, firm evidence for the effectiveness of exclusion diets in improving core autistic symptoms is however lacking. Parents usually exclude foods that they identify as culprits, which can be encouraged as long as it does not lead to dietary inadequacy. The danger in a small minority of families is to take the exclusion too far. In cases of doubt, it is important to involve a paediatric dietician, to ensure the remaining diet is nutritionally adequate. *Food allergies* may also occur: these require paediatric assessment.

BOX 44.2 Case Example

Freda, aged five years, is referred by her general practitioner to the primary mental health worker because she is overweight. Her mother is convinced that she has 'glandular' problems, so the general practitioner also refers her to a paediatrician for endocrine tests. The paediatrician involves the paediatric dietician.

The paediatrician, primary mental health worker and paediatric dietician meet together to pool the results of their assessments. The growth chart shows that Freda is obese. A dietary history establishes that Freda's intake is excessive. The paediatrician does not think endocrine tests are justified. The primary mental health worker has established that both mother and maternal grandmother (who is closely involved with the family, in the absence of any father figure) believe that Freda needs to eat whenever she is distressed or frustrated about anything. Freda says that when she feels sad or unhappy she also feels hungry.

The paediatrician and dietician are running an exercise programme with a local leisure centre for overweight children; Freda and her mother have agreed to join this. The primary mental health worker agrees to work with the family on clearer recognition of emotions and how to respond to them.

Exercise

As with diet, there are various public health measures that can enable or encourage children to take more exercise: these build on a basic target of 60 minutes of physical activity each day, which involves exertion at least twice a week – pushing oneself to the point that one is out of breath, sweaty or aware of one's pulse.[25] Opportunities include: competitive sport and formal exercise; physically demanding activities such as dancing, swimming or skateboarding; or active play such as playing 'it' or kicking a ball around. It is also important to build physical activity into daily life and any regular journeys – for instance by walking, cycling or running up stairs.

In some areas it is possible for doctors to give an exercise prescription – for attendance at a gym or leisure centre. Schools can introduce intensive exercise programmes that help children become more active, leaner and fitter, but it may be difficult to sustain these changes.[26,27]

BOX 44.3 Case Example

> Sarah, aged 14 years, speaks to her general practitioner, initially on her own, about some weight-related teasing she has recently experienced at school. She asks whether she could have some weight-loss pills or a gastric band operation – she has read about both on the Internet. Plotting Sarah's weight and height on a growth chart confirms that Sarah is overweight, but her general practitioner says she is not obese and would certainly not qualify for surgery. He also tells Sarah that diet pills are quite risky and not recommended at her age.
>
> Sarah's mother, who has been in the waiting room, then joins them. She reveals that, as an older teenager, she put on a lot of weight, so she is worried that Sarah will balloon out as well. The general practitioner enquires about diet and exercise. Sarah mentions that she has begun to skip breakfast and occasionally lunch in the hope of losing weight quickly. She and her mother describe a home diet consisting mainly of convenience foods that sounds to the general practitioner as if it is high in saturated fat. The family also lead a sedentary lifestyle with very little exercise.
>
> The general practitioner advises that skipping meals, particularly breakfast, tends to lead to more weight gain and could even develop into an eating disorder. He arranges a one-off appointment with the practice dietician to discuss a suitable diet plan for all the family. He also suggests attempting to incorporate exercise in Sarah's daily routine. Sarah agrees she could walk to school and might even be able to cycle. Sarah and her mother also agree to join the local gym, where a recent advertisement has offered two free sessions of advice from a personal trainer with every new membership. They agree that it would be good for them to support each other in keeping to the exercise programme.

REFERENCES

1 Associate Parliamentary Food and Health Forum. *The Links Between Diet and Behaviour: the influence of nutrition on mental health.* London: HM Government; 2008. Available at:

www.fhf.org.uk/inquiry and www.fhf.org.uk/meetings/inquiry2007/FHF_inquiry_report_diet_and_behaviour.pdf (accessed 6 April 2011).

2 www.rcpsych.ac.uk/mentalhealthinfo/problems/nutrition.aspx

3 www.fabresearch.org

4 Hibbeln JR, Davis JM, Steer C, et al. Maternal seafood consumption in pregnancy and neurodevelopmental outcomes in childhood (ALSPAC study): an observational cohort study. Lancet. 2007; 369: 578–5.

5 Amminger GP, Schäfer MR, Papageorgiou K, et al. Long-chain omega-3 fatty acids for indicated prevention of psychotic disorders. Arch Gen Psychiatry. 2010; 67(2): 146–54.

6 Nemets H, Nemets B, Apter A, et al. Omega-3 treatment of childhood depression: a controlled, double-blind pilot study. American Journal of Psychiatry. 2006; 163(6): 1098–100.

7 Raz R, Gabis L. Essential fatty acids and attention-deficit-hyperactivity disorder: a systematic review. Dev Med Child Neurol. 2009; 51(8): 580–92.

8 Richardson AJ, Montgomery P. The Oxford-Durham Study: a randomized, controlled trial of dietary supplementation with fatty acids in children with developmental coordination disorder. Pediatrics. 2005; 115(5): 1360–6.

9 Sinn N, Bryan J. Effect of supplementation with polyunsaturated fatty acids and micronutrients on learning and behavior problems associated with child ADHD. J Dev Behav Pediatr. 2007; 28(2): 82–91.

10 Vaisman N, Kaysar N, Zaruk-Adasha Y, et al. Correlation between changes in blood fatty acid composition and visual sustained attention performance in children with inattention: effect of dietary n-3 fatty acids containing phospholipids. Am J Clin Nutr. 2008; 87(5): 1170–80.

11 Richardson AJ. Omega-3 for Behaviour, Learning and Mood: what's the real evidence? [presentation given at Food and Behaviour Research Conference, Feeding Success: Why Better Nutrition is Vital for Improving Mental Health and Performance]. Oxford: Saïd Business School; 23 Sep 2010.

12 Richardson, 2005, op. cit.

13 McCann D, Barrett A, Cooper A, et al. Food additives and hyperactive behaviour in 3-year-old and 8/9-year-old children in the community: a randomised, double-blinded, placebo-controlled trial. Lancet. 2007; 370(9598): 1560–7.

14 Schab DW, Trinh NH. Do artificial food colors promote hyperactivity in children with hyperactive syndromes? A meta-analysis of double-blind placebo-controlled trials. J Dev Behav Pediatr. 2004; 25(6): 423–34.

15 Vermiglio F, Lo Presti VP, Moleti M, et al. Attention deficit and hyperactivity disorders in the offspring of mothers exposed to mild-moderate iodine deficiency: a possible novel iodine deficiency disorder in developed countries. Journal of Clinical Endocrinology & Metabolism. 2004; 89(12): 6054–60.

16 DiGirolamo AM, Ramirez-Zea M. Role of zinc in maternal and child mental health. Am J Clin Nutr. 2009; 89(3): 940S–5S.

17 Gesch CB, Hammond SM, Hampson SE, et al. Influence of supplementary vitamins, minerals and essential fatty acids on the antisocial behaviour of young adult prisoners. Randomised, placebo-controlled trial. BJP. 2002; 181: 22–8.

18 Zaalberg A, Nijman H, Bulten E, et al. Effects of nutritional supplements on aggression, rule-breaking, and psychopathology among young adult prisoners. Aggress Behav. 2010; 36(2): 117–26.

19 Field AE, Austin SB, Taylor CB, *et al.* Relation between dieting and weight change among preadolescents and adolescents. *Pediatrics.* 2003; **112**(4): 900–6.

20 Rex D. Understanding and influencing food choices. *Food and Behaviour Research Conference: nutrition for behaviour, learning and mood.* Oxford: Magdalen College; 25 Sep 2009. Figure 44.1 is adapted from his presentation with the permission of David Rex, Specialist Dietician for Health Promoting Schools, NHS Highland.

21 Ibid.

22 www.jamieoliver.com/school-dinners

23 Thaler RH, Sunstein CR. *Nudge: improving decisions about health, wealth and happiness.* New Haven and London: Yale University Press; 2008.

24 McCann, op. cit

25 National Institute for Health and Clinical Excellence. *Promoting physical activity, active play and sport for pre-school and school-age children and young people in family, pre-school, school and community settings* [NICE public health guidance 17]. London: NICE; 2009. Available at: http://guidance.nice.org.uk/PH17/Guidance/pdf (accessed 6 April 2011).

26 Kriemler S, Zahner L, Schindler C, *et al.* Effect of school based physical activity programme (KISS) on fitness and adiposity in primary schoolchildren: cluster randomised controlled trial. *BMJ.* 2010; **340**: c785.

27 van Sluijs EMF, McMinn A. Preventing obesity in primary schoolchildren. *BMJ.* 2010; **340**: c819.

CHAPTER 45

Imaginary friends, voices and psychosis

INTRODUCTION

In adult mental health, the treatment of serious mental illness plays a prominent role. In child and adolescent mental health, serious mental illness occurs in only a small minority of clients, and services are generally dealing with problems of living rather than mental illness.

Many professionals working in mental health are trained to differentiate the normal from the abnormal. However, defining psychosis in children and young people can be fraught with difficulty. Simplistically, characteristic features of psychosis include delusions and hallucinations. Defining a *delusion* as a false, irrefutable belief out of keeping with educational, cultural and social background may work most of the time for adults, but can it be applied to a boy who believes that his transient wish that his younger sister would die led to her developing leukaemia?[1] Similarly, defining a *hallucination* as a sensory perception of something that seems real but would not be accepted as real by anyone else usually works well enough for adults. But does this definition allow for the rich fantasy lives of some children – such as those who have imaginary friends or impersonate them – for whom the distinction between fantasy and reality may appear blurred?

This chapter aims to help child mental health professionals distinguish when childhood fantasy is an expected part of the child's development and when it may be worth worrying about.

THE CONTINUUM OF NORMAL DEVELOPMENT AND PSYCHOSIS

It may be helpful to think of a *continuum*, from what at one end is clearly normal because it occurs so frequently and does not appear to have a negative impact on the child; to what at the other end is clearly psychotic because it matches adult psychotic experience closely.

Fantasy and imagination

Having a very good imagination is often seen as a sign of intelligence or creativity. Being able to engage in sustained imaginative activity may require a temporary withdrawal of consciousness from the world around us. This sort of dissociation is relatively easy for adults, but probably even easier for children. For instance, when

Normal childhood fantasy

Psychotic symptoms with adult-type features

FIGURE 45.1 The continuum from imagination to psychosis

watching a film or reading a novel, we can temporarily suspend our disbelief, suppressing our knowledge that the story and characters are not real: this capacity allows us to enjoy the experience to a greater extent.

Young children are often enchanted by stories and theatrical performances; most will readily engage in extended sessions of make-believe or fantasy play, by themselves or with others. Such a retreat into the world of fantasy helps young children learn to distinguish between fantasy and reality, and generally promotes cognitive and social development. By the age of three years, most children can talk about 'make-believe' or 'pretend', and can distinguish this from what adults regard as reality. Eavesdropping on a conversation may demonstrate this: 'Let's pretend that we're going shopping: I'll be mum and you can be the baby; the shed can be the shop . . .' Children may have more confusion regarding cultural myths such as Father Christmas and the Tooth Fairy, as they are encouraged in these beliefs by adults in a way that blurs the boundaries of the usual adult reality.[2] It is therefore normal for children (and adults) to have a fantasy life that may involve suspension of disbelief, at least for short periods of time. Children who do not appear to be able to engage readily in imaginary play should in fact give rise to more concern. For example, children on the autistic spectrum frequently do not show make-believe play; instead, their play is more likely to include repetitive elements, such as lining up toys excessively or sorting them according to shape, size or colour. Children on the autistic spectrum may also have difficulty distinguishing fantasy from reality, for instance being reluctant to dress up as another person for fear of becoming that person (*see also* Chapter 32 on Autistic Spectrum Disorders).

Children's imaginary creations

Sometimes children engage in fantasy play for extended periods of time. This can be due merely to strong development of imagination skills in the context of normal development; or it can be related to special needs or emotional difficulties. Such children may derive support, reassurance or anxiety relief from their imaginative activities, which may help them process emotionally charged experiences.

Young children aged three to seven years may take on the role of a person or animal (or machine!) whom they impersonate: this can be referred to as **an *imaginary* identity**.[3]

BOX 45.1 Case Example

> At the age of six years, Katherine enjoys for several months imagining herself as Harry Potter. There are occasions when she will respond to a parent or her class teacher only if she is addressed as 'Harry!' This phase passes, and Katherine develops as a very imaginative child who loves listening to stories and enjoys writing her own.

Other young children may have a special toy who appears to have their own likes, dislikes and personality, and with whom the child frequently talks and plays with and may look after. This sort of creation can be termed a ***personified object*** or an ***imaginary companion***.

BOX 45.2 Case Example

At the age of five years, Calie is often accompanied by her toy pony, Minty. Minty always wants to play with Calie and has her own likes, dislikes and feelings. For example, Calie reports that 'Minty likes chewing bubble gum because it makes her mouth exercise'.

More rarely, older children from age seven up even into adulthood may create an elaborate ***imaginary world*** or ***paracosm***.

BOX 45.3 Case Example

By the age of eight, Luke has created an imaginary world over several years called 'Pinwave'. Pinwave has giant spiders and crickets. It once rained pins in this world. There are different parts to Pinwave. Thus Luke reports: 'Lower Pinwave mainly has people with spears because it wasn't as advanced in the medieval times and Upper Pinwave has already developed armour'.

Luke is a very imaginative child who also enjoys writing and producing 'Black Panther' comics. He very much enjoys playing Pinwave with his brother and father and says that it has '. . . made me adventurous'. Luke's paracosm serves the purpose of play and entertainment and as a vehicle for his blossoming imagination.

Paracosms seem to be associated with a heightened imagination. Some famous authors have recalled the imaginary world they created in childhood; for example, C.S. Lewis created 'Animal-land' in his childhood.

More commonly, children may have ***imaginary friends*** (sometimes referred to as ***imaginary companions***).[4,5] Whilst some imaginary friends may develop from a special toy (as referred to above), most imaginary friends are invisible. They may be developed from a story or television character, real people or animals known to the child – or be completely imaginary.

BOX 45.4 Case Example

Rachel, aged six years, has two imaginary friends who are shorter, younger versions of her real friends and have the same names as her friends: Chantelle and Ellen. Rachel teaches her imaginary friends maths and drawing.

> Carmel, a bright and sociable 10-year-old, has created a family of imaginary friends: Tinton and Dubbish, twin boys aged seven; their parents, Betty and Sinjon; later, two baby sisters arrive, Susan and Eileen. Carmel enjoys playing and having adventures with Tinton and Dubbish when there is no one around to play with. She also values being able to talk to them in confidence when things haven't gone so well that day in school: 'At other times, I just play with them and I tell them if something has gone wrong, but then all my emotions just slip away, and I focus on whatever I was talking to them about or playing with them'.

Having an imaginary friend is common, particularly up to the age of seven years: 65% of the population have imaginary friends or report previously having them.[5] Some children in middle childhood (aged seven to 11 years) and adolescents will admit to having an imaginary friend, although in most cases parents and friends are unaware. Children of this age are sometimes reluctant to talk to researchers about their imaginary friends, so there is variation in reporting: 46% of children aged between five and 12 years reported having, or having had imaginary friends, as did 19% of 10 year olds.[6]

Whilst some imaginary friends are described as best friends, others might show naughty or unfriendly characteristics.

BOX 45.5 Case Example

> Antonio, aged five, claims not to like one of his imaginary friends, Ridey, because he is naughty, and Antonio blames Ridey for his own misdeeds when challenged by his parents. At other times, he talks animatedly about the fun he has being naughty with Ridey – hiding and laughing. Antonio is learning both to recognise what is appropriate behaviour and how to regulate his impulses.
>
> Luke – in addition to Pinwave (*see* Box 45.3) – has an imaginary friend called Tom. Luke explains that when someone has annoyed him, he sometimes has a pillow fight with Tom, and that this ends up in a game, which helps him shake off his angry feelings. It is worth noting here that this appears to be an effective strategy: Luke's parents and class teacher comment that he is a friendly, popular and respected member of his class.

Imaginary friends are very much part of normal development and provide a range of positive purposes for the child. These include:
➤ helping him to overcome boredom and loneliness when friends or siblings are not available
➤ a vehicle for imagination, play and entertainment
➤ wish fulfilment
➤ support when things in his life have not gone as he would have liked.

Most imaginary friends show lots of positive qualities. Children describe the friend as showing interest and wanting to play; they are good listeners; they can be trusted with secrets. Even when some imaginary friends are occasionally naughty or unfriendly, often they still seem to serve a positive purpose for the child, helping him to understand and respond to issues in his life. With an imaginary friend who is part of normal development, most children will acknowledge that the imaginary friend is imaginary (though appearing very real to the child), and will regard the imaginary companion as special and mostly helpful to them.

Children with special needs have imaginary friends

Children who have imaginary friends do not form a homogeneous group. Whilst some children with imaginary friends are reported by their parents to be highly imaginative, sociable and early talkers, other children have speech and language difficulties, learning difficulties or a diagnosed condition such as Asperger's syndrome or Down's syndrome. The imaginary friends of such children may meet some or all of the purposes described in the last section, or may serve some more special purposes for the child.

Although there is growing awareness of children with high functioning autism and Asperger's having imaginary friends, their arrival can be disconcerting for parents and teachers. However, a careful developmental history and in depth knowledge of the child's behaviour in different settings can help to distinguish imaginary friends from hallucinations or very early-onset schizophrenia.

From a developmental perspective, imaginary friends can provide important roles for children with Asperger's syndrome or high-functioning autism by helping them to understand and manage social experiences and as a means of trying to make sense of the complexities of human relationships.[7] For example, most children with Asperger's syndrome or high-functioning autism attend mainstream schools where they are generally able to access the curriculum and achieve academic success as well as their typically developing peers. In fact, their good intellectual ability and their social interest may mask the difficulties that they have in trying to establish social relationships and fit in with their peers. Their attempts at trying to socialise can be awkward and they may be frequently rebuffed by their peers. Their realisation of their social isolation and the recognition that they are in some ways different from their peers is a gradual process and usually begins between the ages of six and eight years, potentially causing significant psychological distress.

Clare Sainsbury, an adult with Asperger's syndrome, describes this quite vividly:

> 'Here is one of my most vivid memories of school: I am standing in a corner of the playground as usual, as far way as possible from people who might bump into me or shout, gazing into the sky and absorbed in my own thought. I am eight years old and have begun to realise that I am different in some nameless but all pervasive way. I don't understand the children around me. They frighten and confuse me. They don't want to talk about things that are interesting. I used to think that they were all silly, but now I am beginning to understand that I am the one who is all wrong.'[8]

In response to their social difficulties in establishing friendships with other children, children with Asperger's syndrome or high-functioning autism may adopt compensatory strategies.[9] These strategies can be either negative or positive. Negative psychological strategies include:

➤ internalising negative feelings by developing clinical anxiety or depression (*see* Chapters 20 and 26)
➤ externalising the problem as a solution to feeling different by attributing any difficulties to everyone else, refusing support and denying any social ineptitude. Sometimes behaviour can become intimidating towards other children, for instance through excessive retaliation in response to perceived bullying.

Constructive psychological strategies consist of:

➤ imitation; the child stays on the fringe of peer play activities, watching carefully and mentally noting what other children do. He may re-enact the scenes he has observed in his own play using dolls, soft toys or imaginary friends
➤ escaping into the imagination; a child may develop imaginary worlds or paracosms and/or imaginary friends.

What emerges here is the opportunity to view imaginary friends of children with Asperger's syndrome or high-functioning autism in a positive light, perhaps acting as a self-protective device.

Donna Williams, an adult with Asperger's syndrome, suggests this may be the case when she recalls:

> 'People were forever saying that I had no friends. In fact my world was full of them. They were far more magical, reliable, predictable and real than other children and they came with guarantees. It was a world of my own creation where I didn't need to control myself or the objects, animals and nature, which were simply being in my presence. I had two other friends who did not belong to this physical world: the wisps, and a pair of green eyes which lived under my bed, named Willie.'[10]

Within the context of the expected developmental trajectory of children with Asperger's syndrome or high-functioning autism, imaginary friends may contribute to the attainment of a theory of mind.

BOX 45.6 Case Example

Joanna is a 15-year-old girl with Down's syndrome who attends a mainstream secondary school. Joanna has several imaginary friends who are based on characters from musicals, such as Maria and Tony from West Side Story. Joanna's mother reports that Joanna sometimes seems to interact with her imaginary friends to help prepare her for social situations and life events. She gives an example: Joanna was asked to be a bridesmaid, something that she wanted to do but found anxiety-provoking.

Joanna's mother recalls that Joanna spent much time before the wedding rehearsing the wedding with her imaginary friends. When asked how Joanna had coped on the day, her mother said proudly: 'Brilliantly; she had a big smile on her face all day'.

Sometimes imaginary friends may be more concerning to parents or teachers. For instance, the young person may present as unhappy or anxious and may increasingly withdraw from social situations, preferring to be with his imaginary friends. In such a situation, professional advice should be sought.

Psychotic symptoms

It is worth emphasising that psychotic symptoms do not necessarily indicate mental illness as a cause, and that psychotic mental illness is exceedingly rare before puberty. Hallucinatory experiences are normal during the period between sleep and waking, both on going to sleep and waking up. Seeing or hearing the recently departed loved one is a normal feature of acute bereavement. Auditory hallucinations are common in middle childhood, occurring in 9% of children aged seven and eight years who were asked about the last year in a Dutch study.[11] Such 'voices' were reported by 10% of 12-year-old children asked about the last six months in a British study.[12] This study showed a higher prevalence of a variety of psychotic symptoms in children with an intelligence quotient below 90 and in victims of bullying, particularly if the bullying was chronic and severe.[13] There may be temperamental factors, such as easy suggestibility, determining which children report hearing voices. Obsessional thoughts can be experienced as a separate voice, although assessment will usually reveal that they are a repeated internal monologue, often associated with other features of obsessive-compulsive disorder (*see* Chapter 39).

So the relatively common childhood experience of voices does not necessarily indicate any disorder. Often a voice may be merely one part of the child's mind that expresses a different view from the rest. This may be like the character Jiminy Cricket in 'Pinocchio'. Table 45.1 suggests criteria for professionals to be more or less concerned.

TABLE 45.1 How worried do you need to be about voices?

Which end of the continuum?	Nearer to normal pole	Nearer to psychotic pole
Where is the voice?	Experienced as inside the head or as part of the young person's mind	Experienced as outside the head, as if someone else is really talking
Who is the voice?	A familiar, imaginary figure	A frightening and unknown being; may feel familiar but still be unrecognised
How many voices?	Single	Several

(Continued)

Which end of the continuum?	Nearer to normal pole	Nearer to psychotic pole
Who are the voices talking to?	Exclusively to the young person	At least partly to each other
What are they saying?	Expressing a viewpoint or being a conscience: saying something that the young person himself might think	Command hallucinations telling the young person to kill himself or be violent to others, or be a running commentary about the young person's actions in the third person
Emotional context	The young person appears to accept the presence of the voice, and it is other people who are worried	The young person is scared and uncertain what these experiences are; the young person may feel controlled by the beings he hears

A young person's hallucinations or delusions are commonly due to **organic causes**, such as delirium during high fever, a brain disorder such as encephalitis, or drug ingestion. This may involve prescribed drugs, such as methylphenidate, or non-prescribed drugs, such as ecstasy, cocaine, amphetamines, cannabis or LSD. More rarely, temporal lobe epilepsy can cause a variety of abnormal experiences, including visual or olfactory hallucinations. Visual hallucinations suggest an organic cause more strongly than auditory.

Another cause of hallucinations in any sensory modality is **flashbacks**. These are recurrent memories of a traumatic experience (*see* Chapter 37 on Adjustment Disorder and Post-Traumatic Stress Disorder). The experience may be any sort of trauma, but sexual abuse is a particularly difficult example to assess and manage effectively. The sexual abuse may not have been disclosed, and the memories may be confused and incoherent. Such experiences, whether resulting from past abuse or not, have been described as 'borderline', meaning on the border between neurosis and psychosis. Vivid flashbacks with a realistic quality can occur in adults with a diagnosis of borderline personality disorder. They can often be linked to memories of childhood sexual abuse. The use of this diagnosis in under-18s is potentially rash, in that the personality is not formed until adulthood, so the term 'emerging borderline personality disorder' is generally preferred. This is useful only in so far as it leads to treatment options.

Approaching closer to the psychotic end of the continuum are bizarre experiences in those with **autistic spectrum disorders**, especially Asperger's disorder or high-functioning autism (*see* Chapter 32). The useful function that imaginary friends can play for such individuals is described earlier in this chapter. The increased incidence of psychotic symptoms in autistic individuals may be due to difficulties with:

➤ distinguishing between fantasy and reality
➤ differentiating between internal and external events

➤ abstract thought and the practical use of language (metaphorical statements may be taken literally, resulting for instance in socks being pulled up)

➤ tending to interpret puzzling experiences in a concrete way

➤ expressing emotion appropriately (sad events may be told with a smile, or embarrassment may be expressed with a punch in the chest)

➤ achieving rapport during an interview.

These should be considered before concluding that the person is psychotic.

Psychotic features can occur as a consequence of *severe depressive disorder*. Voices may be making discouraging statements such as:'You're useless' or 'You'd be better off dead'. There may be overpowering feelings, or delusions, of worthlessness or guilt. The content of these experiences is mood-congruent: it is understandable as an extension of other depressive cognitions.

Finally, a first *psychotic episode* presents with phenomena at the psychotic pole of the continuum, including hallucinations and delusions. Auditory hallucinations may have some of the features in the right hand column of Table 45.1. There may be thought echo: hearing one's own thoughts spoken aloud. Spoken thoughts may appear disordered, with links that are difficult to follow or breaks in the train of thought (thought block). Delusions may include:

➤ persecutory delusions: 'People in the street are always saying horrible things about me just out of my hearing'; 'People are out to get me'

➤ grandiose delusions of special powers or missions

➤ delusions of thought interference: that others can hear, read, insert or steal the young person's thoughts

➤ delusions of passivity: that others can control the young person's will, limb movements, bodily functions or feelings.

Providing substance misuse can be excluded, a first psychotic episode may represent the beginning of schizophrenia or bipolar disorder, but either diagnosis is difficult to make on a first episode, and some individuals never have any further episodes. Hence the term 'psychotic episode' is preferred.

ASSESSMENT

Assessment needs to include a history, an exploration of the young person's mental state and an account from other informants (usually parents or carers). Assessments in the early stage of a psychotic illness may reveal more information than subsequent assessments, particularly if medication suppresses the psychotic features or young people may become more reluctant to share their internal experiences.

As indicated above, a *history* should explore possible normalising explanations for any apparently bizarre experiences, before moving through other possibilities on the continuum of psychosis. Substance misuse can cause symptoms at any point on this continuum. As in most interviewing, questions should start open and progress to being more focused if necessary, for instance:

➤ what is worrying you?

➤ what do you think is worrying other people about you?

➤ do you think something funny has been going on?
➤ have you had any unusual experiences?
➤ have you heard any voices that you don't think other people can hear?
➤ have you had any dreams during the day?
➤ what do you think has led to this happening?
➤ could someone be behind any of this?
➤ have the voices suggested you should do anything to yourself?
➤ have the voices told you to do anything to anyone else?

The content of any current hallucinations or delusions should be explored, clarifying risks to self or others. Has there been any actual harm to self or others?

Background factors are also important, such as developmental history, family history, medical history and any previous bizarre experiences.

An exploration of the young person's **mental state** overlaps with the history. Altered consciousness indicates an organic condition and should lead to immediate paediatric referral. Fast or pressurised speech suggests mania. Is mood up, down, all right or flat? Are there obsessions or anxieties? How much insight does the young person have? What do they think is going on?

An **account from informants** should help to clarify the time course and how the young person is being affected by their symptoms. There may be a long delay before presentation to health services, with insidious onset of symptoms. Have there been so-called 'negative symptoms', meaning a deterioration in level of functioning, particularly socially, at school or in terms of prior interests? In adolescence, this is most often due to low mood, the influence of peers or substance misuse. An explanation in terms of psychosis would involve features such as: the development of apathy without low mood; emotional withdrawal with flat affect; a lack of attention to appearance or personal hygiene; or a lack of flowing, spontaneous conversation. Has there been any risky behaviour to self or others? Have there been any changes in behaviour, such as overactivity, disinhibition, sleeplessness or reduced food or fluid intake? A short time course (less than two weeks) and a clearly stressful precipitant indicate a transient psychotic episode, which has a significantly better prognosis than an episode with a long slow onset. Has there been any suspected substance misuse (which the young person may deny)?

MANAGEMENT AND REFERRAL

Management of possible psychosis is simple. The main decision to make is whether the symptoms require further assessment or not. Those presentations clearly at the normal pole of the continuum require reassurance; those at the psychotic pole, or where there is significant doubt, require referral.

Children who have experienced trauma or abuse

Children are not generally referred to clinicians because of their imaginary friends, who are, as described above, usually an aspect of normal, healthy development.

Normal pole   Psychotic pole

Imaginary friends   Imaginary friends in response to abuse
                                        Flashback to previous trauma

Between sleep and waking
                                                          Psychotic episode

High fever   Organic psychosis

Acute bereavement   Emotional disorder   Severe depressive disorder

Note: Substance misuse can cause symptoms on any part of the line

FIGURE 45.2 The continuum between normal development and psychotic symptoms

Imaginary friends can be supportive to children who have emotional problems, for instance because of a difficult family situation; they may in some cases reduce or prevent clinical symptoms.[14]

However, some children referred to clinicians with emotional or psychological difficulties report imaginary companions. One group of significance consists of children who have experienced severe trauma or abuse. Sometimes, these imaginary companions may be supportive, but others on the contrary may be unwelcome, frightening, controlling or may appear to act against the best interests of the child (possibly representing either the child's view of the abuser or the person the child had to become in order to cope with the experience of abuse). The child may show confusion between fantasy and reality.[15] Sometimes, the personality of the imaginary friend may appear to take over the personality of the child (a form of dissociation). Onward referral should be considered for all such cases.

TABLE 45.2 Alarm Bells to look out for in the assessment of possible psychotic experiences

---

Clouding of consciousness suggests the need for paediatric referral. Look for other signs of organic illness, such as fever, headache, sore throat or others. If acutely unwell, make the referral to paediatrics urgent.

Voices commanding suicide or violence suggest the need for urgent psychiatric referral.

Bizarre hallucinations or delusions suggest the need for psychiatric referral.

Very vivid imaginary friends who act against the child's best interests, where there is some reality confusion or dissociation suggest the need for referral for further assessment.

In all cases, try to get a **drug history**.

BOX 45.7 Case Example

When he is nine years old, Paul's mother brings him to the general practitioner at the insistence of his head teacher. Paul has caused great alarm in school by climbing onto a first-floor window ledge as if to jump out, then telling his head teacher that a voice told him to jump out of the window. The general practitioner attempts to engage Paul in conversation, but Paul will not say more than a few words in reply. So his mother agrees to an assessment in specialist CAMHS.

A month later, the general practitioner receives a letter from a consultant child psychiatrist, who reports Paul giving a clear description of his 'voice' as inside his head and expressing ideas of his own. With mother's permission, the consultant child psychiatrist has liaised with the school to obtain their version of events. The threat to jump from a window ledge arose immediately after a fight with another boy, leading to the class teacher telling Paul off. It seemed to the psychiatrist that Paul had wanted to create an effect.

The clinic letter also informs the general practitioner that the family is well-known to various services as struggling to manage financially and emotionally: the three boys and two girls have each given rise to concerns, for instance about their behaviour in school. Paul is the eldest, and seems to elicit the most critical comments from his mother. Family therapy has been offered but not taken up. Mother's current cohabitee has not been prepared to engage with any of the helping services. There has never been sufficient evidence of harm to justify a child protection case conference.

Paul has had some sessions with a CAMHS worker on his own in the past but does not want any more. The consultant child psychiatrist suggests that further involvement of his team is unlikely to achieve much, but he has persuaded Paul's head teacher to arrange additional behavioural support for Paul in school.

BOX 45.8 Case Example

When he is eight years old, Oliver's mother asks to see the community school nurse because she is concerned about Oliver's recent descriptions of a friend called 'Fred', who sometimes tells him to do naughty things. She explains to the community school nurse that Oliver is an only child and seems to have some difficulty making real friends. He rarely asks friends home to play, despite her encouragement to do so. He does not have access to television or computer games at home.

Oliver's mother agrees that the community school nurse can meet Oliver in school to talk to him about Fred. Oliver is very chatty; when they start discussing Fred, Oliver describes him as 'only pretend'. He has known Fred for about three years and has many conversations with him: sometimes Fred suggests things that Oliver might do. Oliver seems reluctant to admit that these might be his own ideas, but eventually agrees with the community school nurse's suggestion that they must come from inside his own head, since that is where Fred comes from.

The community school nurse, with his permission, reports back to Oliver's mother, who is surprised to hear how long Fred has been around. They agree that there is nothing much wrong with her son. They also discuss ways of helping Oliver mix more with children of his own age, such as after-school clubs and sporting activities in the local leisure centre.

ACKNOWLEDGEMENT

We are indebted to Dr Karen Majors, Academic and Professional Tutor of the Institute of Education, University of London and Senior Educational Psychologist for Barking and Dagenham Community Educational Psychology Service; and Dr Anna Calver, Senior Educational Psychologist in the London Borough of Bexley, for sharing their knowledge of and research on imaginary friends to enlarge and improve this chapter, and provide many illuminating brief case examples.

RESOURCE

A book for children

- Burningham J. *Aldo*. London: Red Fox Picture Books; 1993.
  The heroine tells a story about her imaginary rabbit friend, Aldo. This is a book suitable for children of five to eight years who feel alone.

REFERENCES

1 Tiffin PA. Managing psychotic illness in young people: a practical overview. *Child and Adolescent Mental Health.* 2007; **12**(4): 173–86.
2 Taylor M. *Imaginary companions and the children who create them.* Oxford: Oxford University Press; 1999.
3 Harris P. *The work of the imagination.* Oxford: Blackwell; 2000.
4 Majors K. *Children's imaginary companions and the purposes they serve: an interpretative phenomenological analysis* [unpublished doctoral dissertation]. Institute of Education, University of London; 2009.
5 Taylor M, Carlson S, Maring B, *et al.* The characteristics and correlates of fantasy in school-age children: imaginary companions, impersonation, and social understanding. *Dev Psychol.* 2004; **40**: 1173–87.
6 Pearson D, Rouse H, Doswell S, *et al.* Prevalence of imaginary companions in a normal child population. *Child: Care, health and development.* 2001; **27**(1): 13–22.
7 Calver A. *The unicorn who came to stay and other stories . . . mothers' experiences of having a child with autism with an imaginary friend* [unpublished doctoral thesis]. University of East London; 2009.
8 Sainsbury C. *Martian in the Playground: understanding the schoolchild with asperger's syndrome.* 2nd ed. Bristol: Sage Publications (Lucky Duck Books); 2009.
9 Attwood T. *The Complete Guide to Asperger's Syndrome.* London: Jessica Kingsley Publishers; 2008.
10 Williams D. *Nobody Nowhere: the extraordinary autobiography of an autistic.* London: Times Books; 1992.

11 Bartels-Velthuis AA, Jenner JA, van de Willige G, *et al*. Prevalence and correlates of auditory vocal hallucinations in middle childhood. *British Journal of Psychiatry*. 2010; **196**: 41–6.

12 Horwood J, Salvi G, Thomas K, *et al*. IQ and non-clinical psychotic symptoms in 12-year-olds: results from the ALSPAC birth cohort. *BJP*. 2008; **193**: 185–91.

13 Schreier A, Wolke D, Thomas K, *et al*. Prospective study of peer victimization in childhood and psychotic symptoms in a nonclinical population at age 12 years. *Arch Gen Psychiatry*. 2009; **66(5)**: 527–36.

14 Nagera H. The imaginary companion: its significance for ego development and conflict resolution. *Psychoanal Study Child*. 1969; **24**: 165–96.

15 McLewin L, Muller R. Childhood trauma, imaginary companions and the development of pathological dissociation. *Aggression and Violent Behaviour*. 2006; **11**: 531–45.

CHAPTER 46

Sexualised behaviour and gender issues

Introduction

What do you do if a parent asks you whether or not to be worried by the sexualised behaviour her child is showing? Should you be worried about a two-year-old boy who puts on his mother's underwear? How do you know which behaviour is normal, whether it is just exploratory play, whether it is based on observing adult sexual activity or videos, or whether it is a result of participative sexual abuse? Should you reassure and ignore, or should you take it seriously enough to ask social services or a community paediatrician for a further opinion?

It is not always easy to decide whether to be worried about sexualised behaviour or not. Is it just age-appropriate exploration (which Freud believed was normal in under-fives); or does it indicate cause for concern? The nature of the behaviour, the child's associated problems and the level of parental supervision may help decide. It is still only too easy to miss sexual abuse that presents initially as a relatively benign behaviour (*see* Box 46.1); or worry excessively about behaviours that seem to indicate abuse but actually have a more innocent explanation (*see* Box 46.2).

BOX 46.1 Case Example

> Vicky is 13 when her Head of Year becomes concerned when told by the dining room staff that Vicky has grabbed a boy in the crotch. He appeared quite distressed, and a female friend of Vicky's shouted: 'What the f... do you think you're doing?'
>
> The Head of Year interviews Vicky alone in her office. Vicky admits what she did, says she is sorry, and promises not to do it again. Vicky gets up to leave but seems tearful – the Head of Year forms the impression there is something more Vicky wants to say. So she tries to think of an open question that might help Vicky say what she has on her mind. She starts by asking whether everything is all right at home. Vicky says: 'Sort of', and then sits down again.
>
> The Head of Year says: 'Sort of all right and sort of not all right?'
>
> Vicky nods.
>
> 'What's the bit that's not all right?'

Vicky nods.

'What's the bit that's not all right?'

'It's difficult living with a stepbrother.'

'Can you tell me what's difficult about it?'

Eventually, Vicky explains that her 16-year-old stepbrother has been coming into her bed when everyone else in the house is asleep and forcing her to have sex with him.

The Head of Year explains to Vicky that she will have to tell other people about this. Vicky says she just wants it to stop. The Head of Year tells Vicky that she will need to take advice about whom to tell first, but she thinks this will probably include social services and Vicky's mother. She says she will let Vicky know once she has decided.

The Head of Year speaks to the school's safeguarding adviser, who agrees that the Head of Year will have to tell social services but advises against her telling Vicky's mother, as *she* might tell Vicky's father, who might tell his son, and this would prejudice any police investigation. The Head of Year gets hold of Vicky again and explains this to her; she is then able to make the referral to social services, with Vicky's consent, the same day.

BOX 46.2 Case Example

Sandra calls her health visitor in great distress about her three-year-old daughter Amy. Staff at her nursery have asked her to take Amy home after Amy tried to stick a pencil in another child's bottom. The health visitor goes round later the same day. She knows Amy well and asks her what she was trying to do. Amy says she was trying to stick the pencil in the other girl's bum. Undaunted, the health visitor explores this further. Eventually, it emerges that Amy's baby sister was in hospital outpatients earlier the same week, and Amy saw her having a rectal temperature done.

With Sandra's permission, the health visitor calls social services to confirm that she does not need to refer this. As she suspected, a worker at the nursery has already made a referral, stating her concern about the 'sexualised' behaviour and its possible significance. The planned investigation is quickly halted, and the staff at the nursery is reassured. Sandra apologises on Amy's behalf to the other girl's mother, who (fortunately) is able to laugh about it.

A review of normal versus abnormal childhood sexual behaviour emphasises the importance of parental education and discussion about sexual matters, the need for supervision, and the potential influence of increasing media exposure on children's understanding and enactment of sexual behaviour.[1] Boxes 46.3 and 46.4 are taken from this review: they show behaviours which are likely to be normal and those that should give rise to more concern.

BOX 46.3 Examples of sexual behaviours frequently seen in children

Young children (toddler and preschool; early school age)
- Masturbation
- Touching own genitals (behaviour decreases with age)
- Touching mother's breasts (behaviour decreases with age)
- Showing genitals to other children or adults (behaviour decreases with age)

Older children (school age to early adolescence)
- Masturbation (may become more sophisticated)
- Showing interest in the opposite sex
- Asking questions about sex
- Looking at nude photos
- Drawing sexual parts
- Talking about sex
- Using sexual words
- Sex play (touching and/or looking at genitals) between age mates (less than four years age difference) without concerning factors such as force, bribe or threat

BOX 46.4 Sexual behaviours that cause concern

Repeated object insertion into vagina and/or anus
  Age-inappropriate knowledge of sex; for example, knowing how pieces and parts fit together for oral sex, anal sex or intercourse
    Child asking to be touched or kissed in genital area
    Sex play involving one or more of the following:
- Oral-genital contact
- Anal-genital contact
- Genital-genital contact
- Digital penetration of vagina or anus
- Object penetration of vagina or anus
- Four years or greater age difference between children
- Use of force, threat or bribe

Common sexual behaviour in childhood with features that cause concern:
- Increased frequency of the behaviour
- Adults unable to redirect child from the behaviour
- Child's demeanour while exhibiting the behaviour
- Child's talk accompanying the behaviour

The normal behaviours in Box 46.3 are more likely to occur at home than in day care in children aged three to six years: for instance, 33% of children were observed engaging in some form of masturbation at home, but only 5% in day care.[2] Concerning sexualised behaviours of the sort listed in Box 46.4 are more common in children aged 2–12 years who have been sexually abused than in two control groups: CAMHS outpatients and the normal population.[3] Sexualised behaviours that follow sexual abuse have been studied in a longitudinal New Zealand study: this suggests that being a female victim of child sexual abuse before the age of 16 years is likely to lead to the following behaviours in the age range 14–18 years:

➤ early onset sexual activity
➤ teenage pregnancy
➤ multiple sexual partners
➤ unprotected intercourse
➤ sexually transmitted disease
➤ becoming a victim of sexual assault after the age of 16 years.[4]

The recent 'Sexualisation of Young People Review' examines how the increasing use of sexualised images within today's society may be affecting the development and well-being of young people.[5] Whilst sexuality is an important component of physical and mental health, sexualised images in the media are now commonplace and children are exposed to messages and materials from a very young age. Young children do not have the cognitive skills to process and evaluate the persuasive media messages that they are exposed to and have easy access to materials that may not be age appropriate, such as music videos. As children learn vicariously from what they see, they may be adversely affected by this. Concerns about the effects of this on the sexual and emotional development of young people include:

➤ girls may come to value their appearance and accept their treatment as objects of desire
➤ boys may want to be muscular and macho rather than sensitive and emotionally intelligent
➤ friendly relationships between boys and girls may be polluted by premature sexualisation
➤ sexuality may come to be linked with violence, for instance through the increasing exposure of children to pornography
➤ images of super-thin models portrayed as heroines to be emulated may contribute in part to concerns about body image (*see* Chapter 28 on Eating Disorders).

ASSESSMENT, MANAGEMENT AND REFERRAL
Preschool children
Self-stimulation of the genitals is common in both sexes in preschool children. For parents who wish to limit this (there is no need), it usually responds to common-sense techniques such as ignoring or distraction. Alternatively, encouragement to do it in private may be sufficient to satisfy social propriety. Persistent or compulsive masturbation may be due to developmental delay or an overall lack of affection or stimulation. In the absence of such a simple explanation, further investigation (by a social worker or community paediatrician) is advisable.

Dressing in cross-gender clothes is a different issue. Histories taken from adolescents with established habits of cross-dressing suggest that this behaviour commonly starts in the preschool years, often at two or three, and may be inadvertently encouraged by parents, who think it is a joke, and that the little one will grow out of it. An isolated episode may not have much significance; examples include: a two-year-old boy wearing princess slippers at nursery during dressing-up time, or a three-year-old boy with older female siblings joining in with them in having his hair and make-up done. A child may, however, begin to find the behaviour quite rewarding or get fixated about it; for some the act of putting on opposite-gender clothes may be associated with masturbation and sexual satisfaction (from this early age). So parents should be strongly encouraged to put a stop to the behaviour, gently but firmly, before it becomes established. Stopping it at a later age, especially in adolescence or later, may be impossible: it seems that what starts as an exploratory behaviour can become an entrenched pattern with powerful internal reinforcers.

BOX 46.5 Sexual behaviours that cause concern

Nathan, aged four years, is the middle of three boys. His parents have been amother's clothes, but have only just mentioned this to the health visitor, after they found him putting on his mother's panties and rubbing himself on the bed.

The health visitor asks Nathan's parents how they think they could stop this. They explain that they thought he would grow out of it, so they have not done anything about it. The health visitor explains that, if he continued to find such activities pleasurable, Nathan could grow up with a cross-dressing habit that would be difficult to shift. His mother then finds ways to hide her underwear and also supervises Nathan more closely, so that whenever he tries to use her clothes, she distracts him (relatively easily) onto another activity.

Primary school aged (latency) children

Freud believed that sexual impulses were present in the first five years, and then subsided until reawakened in adolescence. Hence the term 'latency'. Sexualised behaviour is less likely to occur in this age group – but when it does, it may be of more concern.

Individual genital play may progress to exploratory play involving others' bodies in situations of children being allowed to play with inadequate supervision. When does play become abuse?

➤ The more the difference in age between children, the more likely the activity is to be abusive. This is more to do with coercion and freely given consent than age itself, and applies to the definition of sexual abuse at any age.

➤ Another dimension is the degree of sexual arousal. Evidence of a child being sexually aroused and obtaining more than just tactile satisfaction should raise questions about how this arousal has developed before adolescence.

➤ Sexualised behaviour involving other children may have been copied, either from actions observed or from actions experienced.

It is worth asking the child whether anyone has touched them in a part of the body where they shouldn't be touched, and whether they have seen anyone doing the things they have been doing. In general, if sexualised behaviour in preadolescents involves other children, it is wisest to refer, probably to social services, to let them make the decision about whether it is abuse or not. They may have information about the family of which you are unaware.

Histories taken from adolescents with **gender dysphoria** (partly or wholly wishing to be the opposite sex) suggest that such thoughts may start in the pre-school or latency years: (boy:) "I felt like a girl in a boy's body"; (girl:) "I was always doing boyish things and wanted to be in boys' clothes." Unlike the cross-dressing mentioned above, this seems to be a pattern of internal thoughts and feelings that develops gradually into observable behaviours, and is therefore not so susceptible to prevention or early intervention.

Education about appropriate and inappropriate forms of touching or other sexual contact may be useful in this age group. This can involve the use of dolls, drawing or painting. This sort of work may be done by a therapeutic social worker working within a specialist Tier 2/3 CAMHS, but others may be willing to take on this task, which does not require specialist training.

Adolescence

Masturbation is virtually universal amongst adolescent boys, but probably occurs in a smaller percentage of girls. Some learning disabled or autistic youngsters lack a sense of public propriety, and need to be taught where they can and can't masturbate. This can be helped by visual aids, symbols or pictures that explain this (*see* Figures 46.1 and 46.2).[6] Occasionally, it forms a crude sexual overture by a socially naïve or learning disabled boy to one or more girls, who complain, so that the boy is accused of indecent exposure. Recognising his lack of social skills leads to a more sympathetic response than considering him perverted.

Experimental sexual behaviour amongst adolescents should be consensual. Problems arise when it isn't. An arbitrary age gap of five years is used in some definitions of sexual abuse, but it is really the degree of mutual willingness that is important. A variety of circumstances may lead girls to become involved against their will in sexual acts with boys, but other combinations can occur. For instance, a promiscuous girl may involve a naïve boy, who may be too ashamed to say no, in some sort of sexual activity. He may feel just as ashamed as a girl who has been raped, or a boy who has been buggered, and have just as much difficulty telling anyone.

In Scotland, children under 12 cannot consent. In England, the **Sexual Offences Act 2003**[7] has made any penetrative sex with a person under the age of 13 years equivalent to rape. Between 13 and 16 years, sexual relations are still technically illegal, but unlikely to incur any police involvement providing consent has been freely given. *Working Together* states that there is a presumption of reporting anyone under 13 having a sexual relationship to social services or the police. It does **not** advocate mandatory reporting.[8] Each case should be considered on its merits,

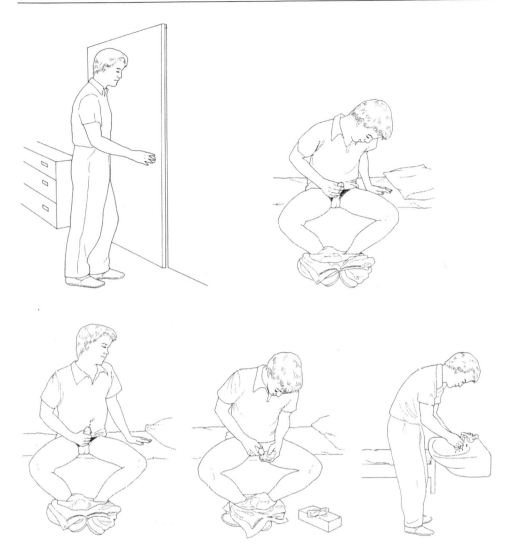

FIGURE 46.1 Masturbation picture story
(Caution: contains explicit images)

taking into account behaviour, living circumstances, maturity, serious learning disabilities, and other factors affecting vulnerability. Information on under-13s should usually be shared, but if a decision is made not to disclose there should be discussion with a named or designated child protection professional, with a record of the decision stating the reasons.[9] (*See also* Chapter 12 on Child Abuse and Safeguarding.)

Indications for therapy. An abusive episode such as a rape may be revealed to a professional some years after the event. The victim's account should make it clear whether the episode was consensual or not. She should be encouraged to report the incident to the police or social services, even if it happened a long time ago. This will enable a check on whether any other children may be at risk. However, the young person may have the capacity to refuse (*see* Chapter 43), in which case she can veto the involvement of other agencies. If she requests someone to talk to (make sure it is the young person and not just the parent making this request), she will need to be referred to victim support, an adolescent counselling service or a specialist CAMHS.

<u>Private</u>
Being in **PRIVATE** means being on my own.

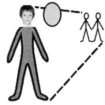

I have a place I can go to be in private, it is my bedroom.

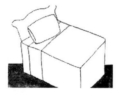

If I want to masturbate I will go to my bedroom. My bedroom is the best place to be in private. I will only masturbate in my bedroom in private.

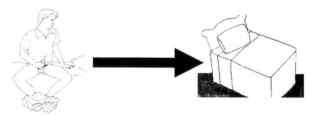

This is the correct way to behave, it is the grown up way to act

FIGURE 46.2 The importance of being private

BOX 46.6 Case Example

A 12-year-old girl, Judy, comes to see the community school nurse in her school drop-in clinic to ask how she could get hold of some contraceptives. The community school nurse is rather alarmed, but tries to hide this from Judy. Judy says she will not explain why she needs them, because she thinks the community school nurse will probably have to tell someone. The community school nurse admits that Judy is partially right: she would have to tell someone else if she thought Judy (or anyone else) was coming to harm. The community school nurse gives Judy some condoms and asks her to come back the following week to discuss going on the oral contraceptive pill.

Rather to the surprise of the community school nurse, Judy does come back. The community school nurse has in the meantime discussed an approach with her local safeguarding nurse: she asks Judy to suppose she is asking on behalf of a friend. If the friend were having sex with an older boy, would Judy be worried about this? Judy says the hypothetical friend knows what she is doing; that as long as the boy is only a bit older and the friend does not feel any pressure, Judy thinks what she is doing is probably all right. But she knows the friend's parents would not approve, and the boy's parents think his girlfriend is the same age as him. Judy still wants to get the pill for her friend, as she has heard that condoms sometimes split, and her friend really does *not* want to become pregnant. The community school nurse says she will need to discuss this with a doctor, and gets Judy's permission to have a discussion with Judy's general practitioner and a community paediatrician: but Judy will not allow the community school nurse to discuss her situation, even anonymously, with social services, as she has a friend who was interviewed by a social worker with no outcome other than a lot of upset for her family. The community school nurse carefully writes up the notes, including her discussion with the safeguarding nurse.

As the community school nurse expected, the general practitioner is not happy to prescribe the pill for a 12 year old. The community paediatrician is the designated doctor for safeguarding and says she might be prepared to do so if Judy would agree to see her, and if it were clearly for Judy rather than her fictional friend. The community school nurse is able to bring Judy to a special appointment with Dr Shelley, who goes through the Gillick checklist (*see* Chapter 43). She tries to persuade Judy to inform her parents, but Judy refuses. She explores with Judy whether she is being exploited, and it seems that Judy is emotionally and intellectually mature enough to give informed consent to a sexual relationship. Judy seeks further reassurance that social services will not be informed.

Dr Shelley decides that it is more important to prevent pregnancy than inform the authorities. She emphasises the medical risks of the pill, and the need to use condoms as well to prevent sexually transmitted diseases. She gives Judy a long-lasting contraceptive injection, which Judy thinks would be safer than having to remember a pill every day (and risk her parents finding the box). Judy and the community school nurse agree on follow-up arrangements. Dr Shelley carefully records in her notes the reasoning behind her decision.

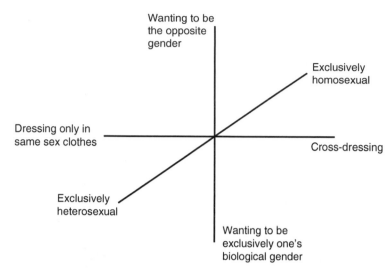

FIGURE 46.3 Three almost independent (orthogonal) axes of gender attitudes

Gender issues

Gender issues can be regarded as being on three orthogonal (partially independent) axes (spectra):

➤ wearing gender appropriate clothes or cross-dressing
➤ gender euphoria or dysphoria
➤ sexual orientation.

Although there is some overlap between these three, it is helpful to think of them as largely independent (*see* Figure 46.3). Confusion may, however, easily arise. For instance, a girl who believes she is really a boy may regard sexual activity with other girls as heterosexual rather than implying she is a lesbian. A boy who finds cross-dressing sexually exciting may find himself more sexually aroused with his girlfriend when he has cross-dressed. A boy who has a well-developed alternative persona as a girl may nevertheless have sexual relationships exclusively with girls.

In early childhood, it is usually possible to shift habits early in their development (*see* Box 46.5 above); but once habits are well-established, it is important to be as accepting as possible – for instance, of cross-dressing behaviour or any conviction of being the opposite gender. Attempts to get the behaviour (or worse still the feelings) to stop once they are well-established are likely to antagonise the young person and make adequate assessment and therapeutic engagement more difficult.

BOX 46.7 Sexual behaviours that cause concern

> Jenny, an eight-year-old girl, has always been a tomboy. She has recently told her mother that she really wants to be a boy rather than a girl. While she does not dislike girls, she explains that she just feels more like a boy.

Her mother is not very surprised to hear this. From an early age, Jenny has only ever wanted to wear trousers in grey, navy or red (boy colours), has always wanted her hair cut short and has always preferred to be out playing on the estate with the boys, kicking balls around, building dens and climbing trees. Since starting at middle school, Jenny has insisted on having boys' trousers to wear to school and boys' tracksuit bottoms out of school; she also insists on going to the barber's rather than the hairdresser's to have her hair cut.

Young people with a *gender identity disorder* often report feeling from an early age that their *real* gender is the opposite of their birth gender (*see* Box 46.7). They identify more strongly with children of the opposite sex, preferring to play with them and dress like them. With the onset of puberty and adolescence, their discomfort at being in the wrong body intensifies, leading in many cases to deliberate self-harm. Many try to keep their true feelings hidden from others for as long as possible, but 'coming out' often provides a sense of relief for the young person – although this may be extremely difficult for parents, who may experience a sense of loss and go through a grieving process. Information, advice and referral to specialist CAMHS at this stage can be extremely helpful.

Initial assessment may result in onward referral to a specialist (Tier 4) clinic. Referral of a young person with a gender identity disorder or gender dysphoria can be made at any age, if the young person and parents want full assessment and specialised treatment. After further specialist assessment, treatment may be offered in the form of psychological therapies and even pharmacological interventions such as hormone-blockers to suppress puberty. Gender reassignment surgery may be offered after the age of 18.

It is not only the child's own feelings about gender that may have an impact, but also the child's feelings about *parental gender issues* (*see* Box 46.8 below). A child who has grown up with a transsexual parent or one with a gender identity disorder may experience some problems as he becomes increasingly aware of his parent's behaviour and how this is different from that of other parents or society's norms. While cross-dressing – temporarily converting to an alternative persona – is compatible with harmonious family life, there are potential problems.[10] These may include:

➤ changes in family circumstances
➤ the adjustment of the other parent
➤ the adjustment of other family members
➤ comments of neighbours, peers at school or others in the community
➤ the child's adjustment to the parental issues themselves and the reaction of others to them.

People going through gender reassignment are usually offered some support and advice as part of the process; other family members may seek support in their own right.

BOX 46.8 Sexual behaviours that cause concern

Marie, the mother of three children – Toby (aged seven years), Phoebe (aged five years) and Thomas (aged three years) – approaches the community school nurse at a drop-in clinic. Ten months ago, Marie's husband (who fathered the children) decided to opt for gender reassignment, having been secretly attending a specialist clinic for some time. Marie was so shocked by this decision that she immediately asked her husband to leave the family home. Since then, the children have hardly seen their father at all, but regular contact arrangements have recently been agreed.

Marie has been seeing a health centre counsellor regularly and has found this very helpful. Partly at the counsellor's suggestion, she has come to discuss how to understand what the children are going through, so she can better meet their needs.

The children have been talking about daddy wanting to be a woman, having seen him recently in female apparel and make-up. They have started asking their mother why he can't still live with the family. Marie has found it hard to know how to explain anything.

Marie and the community school nurse discuss how much the children are likely to be aware of and what they should be told. They agree on a fairly simple but honest explanation that Marie can give the children. This involves saying that mummy was happy to live with daddy when he was a man, but daddy now wants to be a woman. Mummy doesn't want to live with a woman, so mummy and daddy can't live together anymore. They agree that the initial conversation should be with all three children and kept short, with the option of questions immediately afterwards or later, and the possibility for further discussion with each child separately, at an age-appropriate level.

The community school nurse meets with Marie again two weeks later. Marie recounts that the children seem to have more or less accepted her explanation, but that Toby remains very angry with her decision to make his father leave; Phoebe and Thomas seem much less so. Marie reflects that she can accept Toby's anger at the departure from home of his father but hopes that regular contact may help him with this, as well as the opportunity for continued discussions between mother and son.

Marie says she would like to continue meeting with the community school nurse about once a month, as well as seeing her own counsellor, since she wants to keep her own needs and the children's needs separate. The community school nurse affirms that this seems very sensible and caring.

During the subsequent conversations between Marie and Toby, it emerges that he is worried that he will turn into a girl when he is older. After discussing this with the community school nurse, Marie tells Toby that she cannot predict the future, and it is possible that Toby may want to become a girl, but it will be up to him to decide. She also explains that his father spent several years thinking about whether or not he really wanted to become a woman, initially without telling mummy anything about it. Toby finds it difficult to discuss this with his father, but eventually Marie persuades her ex-husband to give Toby some explanation himself.

Phoebe is able to tell her mother that things have been a bit difficult at school for Toby and herself. Although both children (and Marie!) have tried to keep things secret, some of the Year 6 children have somehow found out that their father is hav-ing a sex change and have told some of the younger children that he is a 'hermaph-rodite', although none of the children in school seems to know what this word means. Marie and the community school nurse arrange to see the head teacher to explain what is happening and ask for her help. The three of them meet after school with both class teachers (Toby's and Phoebe's). They decide that an announcement in whole school assembly would probably *not* be a good idea, but that each class teacher will encourage a simple discussion in class, after planning alone with Marie and each of the two older children what they are going to say.

Various other issues come up that Marie and the community school nurse are able to discuss, prior to Marie helping the children understand and accept what is going on. Although Marie's relationship with her ex-husband remains fraught, she becomes able to talk sensibly with him about the children's needs, and all three chil-dren gradually become more accepting of the situation.

BOX 46.9 Practice Points on sexualised behaviour

Cross-dressing in toddlers should be gently but firmly discouraged.

Masturbation is usually normal behaviour; it is generally its social acceptability that is the issue.

Sexualised play between pre-adolescent children may be normal, although it sug-gests a worrying lack of supervision. Any sexual activity involving other children has the potential to be abusive and should usually be referred to social services.

Sexualised activity between adolescents should be regarded as a form of abuse if one party experiences it as coercive, or if one party is under 13 (or age 12 in Scotland).

Adolescent cross-dressing or gender dysphoria should be accepted with as much understanding as possible.

RESOURCES

- **Brook** for young people gives all sorts of advice about sexuality and sexual relationships for under-25s. www.brook.org.uk
- **The Queer Youth Network** is a national organisation run by and for young people with ques-tions about their gender and sexuality. www.queeryouth.org.uk
- **Mermaids** supports young people up to the age of 19 who are trying to cope with gender identity issues and their families and carers. www.mermaidsuk.org.uk
- **The Gender Identity Research and Education Society** provides information for young peo-ple with gender variance and their families. www.gires.org.uk
- **The Gender Trust** supports all those who are affected by gender identity issues. Various informative leaflets can be downloaded, including *Gender Dysphoria – An Introductory Guide for GPs and Health Professionals* at: www.gendertrust.org.uk

- Department of Health. *Transgender Experiences – information and support for trans people, their families and healthcare staff.* London: Department of Health; 2007. Available at: www.dh.gov.uk/en/Publicationsandstatistics/Publications/PublicationsPolicyAndGuidance/DH_081579 (accessed 6 April 2011).

REFERENCES

1 Hornor G. Sexual behavior in children: normal or not? *J Pediatr Health Care.* 2004; **18**(2): 57–64.

2 Larsson I, Svedin CG. Teachers' and parents' reports on 3- to 6-year-old children's sexual behaviour – a comparison. *Child Abuse & Neglect.* 2002; **26**(3): 247–66.

3 Friedrich WN, Fisher Jl, Dittner CA, *et al.* Child sexual behaviour inventory: normative, psychiatric and sexual abuse comparisons. *Child Maltreatment.* 2001; **6**(1): 37–49.

4 Fergusson DM, Horwood LJ, Lynskey MT. Childhood sexual abuse, adolescent sexual behaviours and sexual revictimisation. *Child Abuse & Neglect.* 1997; **21**(8): 789–803.

5 Papadopoulos L. *Sexualisation of Young People.* London: Home Office; 2010.

6 Brook. *Picture Yourself: a sex education resource for people with learning difficulties. Living Your Life: 68 photocopiable worksheets.* London: Brook; out of print. Available from Steve Clarke, Senior Clinical Nurse in Children's Learning Disability, Dorset Healthcare NHS Foundation Trust, Oakcroft, 42 Gravel Hill, Wimborne, Dorset, BH21 1RR.

7 Sexual Offences Act 2003. Available at: www.opsi.gov.uk/Acts/acts2003/ukpga_20030042_en_1 (accessed 6 April 2011).

8 HM Government. *Working together to safeguard children: a guide to interagency working together to safeguard and promote the welfare of children.* 2006. Previously available at: www.everychildmatters.gov.uk/workingtogether

9 General Medical Council. *Zero to 18 Years: guidance for all doctors.* London: General Medical Council; 2007.

10 http://en.wikipedia.org/wiki/Grayson_Perry

CHAPTER 47

Stealing

INTRODUCTION

Stealing is not necessarily a mental health problem, but may be a moral or legal problem and is a problem for the victim of theft.

Why would a parent seek professional advice about her child's stealing? Perhaps she has been pressurised by others to ask for help, or perhaps she has found that nothing she has tried works, and is therefore desperate for some input from outside the family. Police, courts or the local Youth Offending Team may be involved. Shoplifting is very common in young people, implying that it could almost be regarded as normal. It may sometimes be associated with mental health problems in the young person, such as ADHD or a depressive disorder; or with some difficult relationships within the family; or be a means of obtaining money for drugs or alcohol.

ASSESSMENT

There are various patterns of theft. We have divided these into six types, but other divisions could be made, and the categories may overlap in individual cases.

➤ *Marauding* – A group of children or young teenagers go shoplifting together, or raid unattended premises. This is essentially a recreational activity, on a par with group truancy, trespassing or vandalism. There may not be much wrong with the children or their families except that they are poorly supervised.

➤ *Proving* – A teenager steals something which can be exhibited to friends and elicit their admiration. Such an activity is usually fuelled by poor self-esteem or difficulties with peer relationships. Something has to be done to enhance prestige within the group and help establish some self-worth: in this situation, stealing can sometimes be part of an initiation task that is necessary for a young person to be allowed into a specific peer group. Poor self-esteem of the sort which leads to such behaviour may be due to a number of factors, including family scapegoating (*see* Chapter 8 on Family Issues), poor academic ability, clumsiness, short stature, delayed puberty or past traumatic brain injury.

➤ *Comforting* – This applies to the child who steals money from home as a way of compensating for a lack of parental attention, approval or love. The money may be hoarded or spent privately, often on seemingly insignificant things such as sweets: the main motive for the theft seems rarely to be what is bought. This pattern of repeated stealing of parental cash may be a way of (consciously or unconsciously) punishing the parents for not providing a perceived need – or, to put it another way, the child may be trying to communicate how she feels about what she is not being given. It usually indicates a poor relationship between parents and child – and will probably do nothing to improve it. The parents of such children may appear to professionals to be rejecting towards the child.

Solitary theft outside the home, with hoarding of the booty, may also be a form of comforting. A child who steals from other children at school may be expressing a similar need for personal comfort in the face of hostility or rejection from other children. Teenage girls who steal babies or pets are commonly looking for something to look after in order to compensate for feeling uncared for themselves (some may have their own child for this reason); a few may be compensating for a recent termination of pregnancy.

An apparent hybrid between proving and comforting occurs when the child steals money from home, then buys sweets which can be handed round at school in order to buy friendship.

➤ *Secondary* – Some children steal because they have been directly instructed to by a parent, to pay off a bully, due to poverty, or out of necessity while running away.

➤ *Addiction* – Stealing can become necessary to finance an addiction, for instance to street drugs or arcade machines.

➤ *Associated with mental health problems* – Since stealing is one of the symptoms of *conduct disorder*, and lying (to get out of trouble) often accompanies stealing and is also on the conduct disorder symptom list, the association of stealing with antisocial behaviour is tautologous. It seems often to be linked with *ADHD*, perhaps partly because impulsivity and thrill-seeking lead to rash, thought-free acts, of which stealing is a common example (others include driving away others' cars or cycling too fast downhill). Stealing may occur in *depressive disorder*, perhaps driven by a desire to alleviate depressive feelings by getting a thrill or an extra possession – this could be seen as similar to comforting.

BOX 47.1 Case Example

Maryam's parents are so cross with her for stealing cash at home that they ground her for three weeks: she is 13 years old. For cultural reasons, Maryam's mother experiences the theft as bringing great shame upon the family.

Maryam confides to the community school nurse in the school drop-in clinic that she is very fed up with her mother and stepfather, who appear to be far more interested in their new baby than in her. The community school nurse asks Maryam whether she would like her to talk to Maryam's mother, and Maryam says she would not: she just wants someone to talk to on her own about her situation.

Maryam continues to see the community school nurse in the drop-in clinic. She agrees with her that the main reason for her stealing relates to how she feels she is being treated at home, rather than because of the make-up she was able to buy with the money. Using role-play, they rehearse how Maryam might be able to talk to her mother alone and explain how she feels; Maryam finds this so difficult that it requires several sessions. Eventually, Maryam succeeds in finding a calm way of explaining her feelings to her mother in the role-play and is able to enact this at home.

To Maryam's great surprise, her mother bursts into tears and says she has been afraid Maryam might be feeling like that, and it makes her feel really guilty. Mother and daughter build on their newfound closeness, and the stealing does not recur.

BOX 47.2 Case Example

Steven, aged seven years, is the third of five children in a family with a variety of social problems. Because of significant behaviour problems at school, he has been diagnosed with ADHD, and a trial of medication shows significant improvement in school. Unfortunately, his parents are not able or willing to travel to the clinic, and they also periodically decide things are better, so stop the medication. His management therefore requires regular home visits by the ADHD specialist nurse. He enjoys showing her the birds in the family's aviary.

Steven's parents are concerned about his compulsive stealing; he takes whatever he can from the neighbourhood and school, and is not usually caught. Steven cannot give a reason for his stealing: most of the stuff he takes he hoards in his room. The ADHD specialist nurse notices that he seems to steal far more when he is off medication, so realises that it is probably important for Steven to be supported in taking it regularly. She continues to do this until he is 14 years old, when he decides he does not want to take it anymore.

Subsequently, the police gradually become aware of the repetitive nature of Steven's thefts: he becomes involved in the criminal justice system and requires support from the Youth Offending Team. He narrowly avoids a custodial sentence.

MANAGEMENT

Does the stealing fall into the *secondary* category above? If it is prompted by a straightforward motive such as greed or parental instruction, then there may be no role for a mental health professional. In the first instance however, if the stealing is reported to authorities, it is likely that the police and possibly the local Youth Offending Team may be involved. In the case of parental instruction, running away or poverty, social services may need to do an assessment with regard to child protection issues.

Is there any reason to think the child *depressed* or *addicted*? Depression is likely to need further assessment and treatment, particularly if moderate or severe (*see* Chapter 26). Addiction is treatable only if there is some motivation to change, which is rare in teenagers. In some cases, the criminal justice system may help, either through the support of a worker from the Youth Offending Team, or through the threat of punishment by the courts. Referral to a substance misuse team may help. A young person stealing to finance an addiction to gambling or arcade games can be referred to a psychologist or cognitive-behavioural therapist for habit-reduction strategies.

Otherwise, the key issue is whether the theft took place inside or outside the home. *Marauding* theft requires parents to increase their supervision of the young person. They should know where he is and whom he is with all the time.

When stealing is identified, the young person should be helped to return the items or make restoration to the victim including an apology. Parents are often reluctant to do this if it will involve returning to a shop and possible prosecution.

From a management point of view, solitary theft outside the home can be split into two categories. If the goods are hoarded, it should be treated as *comforting* (see next paragraph). If they are shown to others or given away, assume a *proving* motive in the first place. The young person can be helped to find other ways of gaining approval from others. This may include support from a youth worker, involvement in structured activities after school and at weekends, social skills training, counselling from a voluntary agency or support from a Connexions personal adviser.

BOX 47.3 Case Example

Kyle, aged 13 years, is caught shoplifting on several occasions on closed circuit television. The police discuss this with his mother, who also discusses it with his school. It emerges that he has been stealing food and compact discs, which he then gives to peers at school whom he wants to be his friends. He was born prematurely, was short for his age, has always been clumsy and is having help in school for literacy difficulties – so has always tended to feel a bit different from his peers.

The police give Kyle a caution and explain that they will take him to court if he is caught again. The head of pastoral care in his school encourages Kyle to take part in after-school activities, and he chooses two afternoons per week that appeal to him. The Connexions personal adviser attached to his school knows the youth worker at Kyle's local youth club, who agrees to help Kyle attend on Friday evenings. His mother enrols him in a karate class on Saturday mornings. His father promises him a drum kit for his 14th birthday if he stops stealing, which fortunately he does.

Stealing from home is likely to be *comforting.* Comforting stealing can be difficult to treat, but a common-sense intervention is to tell parents to lock money and valuables away (they are often curiously reluctant to do so, citing the need for trust). Also, check if the young person is receiving enough pocket money. Communication within the home may need to be improved, and a more positive atmosphere engendered. Parents may need support to emphasise the positive aspects of the young person's behaviour, to 'catch him being good' and to develop forms of praise and rewards that improve self-esteem and family relationships (*see* the *praise* and *tangible reward* sections of Chapter 13).

REFERRAL

Referral to specialist CAMHS may be useful only if the stealing behaviour is seen as a symptom of a mental health problem, such as depression or ADHD. When there are other explanations for stealing, other agencies are likely to be more appropriate, such as the local Youth Offending Team or social services; there may be local parenting support programmes specifically designed to help parents of young people who offend. Consultation, if available, with a primary mental health worker or specialist CAMHS may help to identify which service is most appropriate in the first instance.

BOX 47.4 Practice Points for managing stealing

Is the child *marauding*? If so, encourage parents to provide more supervision.

Is the child *proving*? If so, clarify any causes of low self-esteem, arrange sociable activities and find ways for parents to bolster his self-image.

Is the child *comforting*? If so, there may be a need for some form of counselling for the child or caregivers.

Is the child stealing due to poverty or parental encouragement (*secondary* stealing)? If so, social measures may be necessary, or it may not be possible to help.

Is the young person stealing to finance *drug use*? If so, try to involve your local substance misuse service.

Is the young person addicted to *arcade games*? If so, will the young person engage with a cognitive-behavioural therapist?

Does the child have *ADHD*? Has this been assessed or treated yet?

Is the young person *depressed*? If so, referral to specialist CAMHS may be necessary.

CHAPTER 48

Referral to specialist CAMHS and other agencies

INTRODUCTION

Not all child and adolescent mental health problems can be managed by Tier 1, universal services or primary care alone. Indications for referral to Tier 3 specialist/multidisciplinary CAMHS include:

➤ the child's symptoms are too serious or severe for primary care professionals to help
➤ when symptoms are still causing significant impairment despite intervention from primary care professionals
➤ the young person or parent(s) request more specialist assessment or treatment.

It can be helpful if possible to discuss the referral in advance with a primary mental health worker or other Tier 2 worker to explore:

➤ alternative referral pathways
➤ how best to phrase the referral letter
➤ how best to explain the need for referral to the young person and carers.

Indications for referral

Common areas for further assessment include:

➤ depression
➤ eating disorders
➤ autistic spectrum disorder
➤ ADHD
➤ obsessive-compulsive disorder
➤ phobias or other anxiety disorders
➤ post-traumatic stress disorder
➤ post-abuse management
➤ self-harm
➤ psychosis
➤ tics that are causing distress
➤ severe behaviour concerns.

Explanation

Prior to making any referral it is very important to explain as much as you can to the young person and family about the reasons for referral and what they might expect, otherwise they may not attend any appointment offered, or may be taken aback when they are later greeted by an unexpected mental health professional. It is therefore helpful to know as much as possible about the service to which you are referring. The explanation should include:

➤ the rationale or need for the referral
➤ the reason for choosing that particular agency
➤ the range of people the young person or family might be asked to see, together or separately
➤ which bits of what they are likely to experience may repeat what the family has already been through, and which bits are likely to be new experiences
➤ practical aspects, such as:
  — how to get to the new clinic
  — where to park if going by car
  — how long the first appointment is likely to last
  — whether they are likely to have any choice about the time of day or the day of the week for the initial or subsequent appointments.

The more thorough the explanatory discussion, and the more the concerns of the young person and family can be anticipated, the more likely they will be to attend the first and subsequent appointments, and so make full use of the service on offer.

Local service information leaflets or information sheets can be a helpful addition to this verbal explanation. If there is no locally produced version, then there are nationally produced leaflets on specialist CAMHS services.[1,2,3]

HOW BEST TO MAKE A REFERRAL

A referral should be made in writing unless considered very urgent. For instance, following an overdose, a telephone referral to Accident and Emergency or paediatrics may be more appropriate.

Different services will have different criteria about who can make a referral. Often the family members will approach their general practitioner for a referral to specialist CAMHS, but other Tier 1 staff may also be able to make direct referrals themselves (there is an absurd amount of geographical variation).

Ideally, the general practitioner, as the hub of the network of health professionals around any patient, should be kept informed, as should other professionals involved with the presenting problems, such as a social worker or educational psychologist. Sometimes, family members may want the referral to be kept confidential from one or more other professionals – this wish should be taken into consideration but not necessarily dictate the professional's actions. For instance, it would be inappropriate not to inform an allocated social worker of the referral of a family in which the children are on the Child Protection Register. There needs to be a very good reason for *not* informing the general practitioner: one example is if one of the receptionists is related to the child being referred (it may be possible to get round this by using secure e-mail).

What to include in a referral letter

As much as possible of the following information should be included in written referrals.

➤ The young person's name and date of birth.
➤ Relevant family members – usually this will include those living with the young person and important absentees, such as a separated parent.
➤ The nature of the concern.
➤ Who is most concerned?
➤ How long has there been concern? Has it developed over time?
➤ Why is the referral now?
➤ Any pertinent factors in the developmental history, such as major illnesses or separations.
➤ Any pertinent factors in the family history, such as divorce, bereavement, house moves or family health problems.
➤ Interventions that have already been tried and their outcome.
➤ Other professionals involved with the family.
➤ The young person's school, with any relevant educational concerns.
➤ The young person's current medication.
➤ The attitude to the referral of the young person and carer(s).

Many general practitioners are able to include a software-generated summary of the young person's current medication and past reasons for visiting the health centre.

REFERRAL TO WHOM?

As an alternative source of help, or in addition to referring to specialist CAMHS, consider involving the following agencies or procedures.

➤ The *Common Assessment Framework* (CAF) is intended to become a national basis for working with families (in England).[4] It provides a framework for professionals to share information, and can form the basis of a comprehensive assessment of all the child's needs, including mental health needs. Many areas are now using the Common Assessment Framework as a prelude to involving social services (or in some areas the NSPCC) in concerns about a child in need and in all but the most severe cases of child abuse.[5]
➤ *Children's centres* may house many of the services set up to help under-fives and their families.
➤ *Information shops* can provide locally tailored information about what support is available. In some areas, services provided by health, education and social services are provided together in a '*one-stop shop*' which should in principle be much more convenient for both families and professionals.
➤ *Educational Psychology Services* help schools, children and parents when there are concerns about educational need or school behaviour. They can be uni-disciplinary (consisting only of educational psychologists) or multidisciplinary

(including for instance social inclusion pupil support workers, assistant psychologists or even social workers). Access is usually through school, but in some areas referral from other sources is allowed.

➤ *Connexions* offers support, counselling and careers advice to young people aged 13–19 years. The local office and contact number are easy to find on the Internet.[6] Connexions should be available everywhere, but in practice, the availability of personal advisers, and how referrals are prioritised, varies geographically.

➤ *Voluntary agencies providing counselling services* – These vary in name and function, for instance in the age range of young people they accept, the duration of counselling offered and whether there is individual or group counselling or both.

➤ *Other voluntary agencies* may provide a variety of services oriented to young people, such as for instance finding accommodation for the homeless.

➤ *Substance misuse services for young people* – This is a specific service for young people with drug and alcohol related concerns: the exact name varies geographically.

➤ *Paediatrics* – In many areas, paediatricians (usually in the community but sometimes in hospital) may provide stigma-free services quicker or more acceptably than specialist CAMHS (or in some cases *in the absence* of a service provided by specialist CAMHS). Services provided by paediatrics may include: assessment and treatment of ADHD (*see* Chapter 31), assessment of autistic spectrum disorder (*see* Chapter 32), assessment and treatment of dyspraxia or sensory difficulties (with paediatric occupational therapy – *see* Chapter 34), and assessment and treatment of tic disorders (*see* Chapter 25).

➤ *Relateen* is a branch of Relate that is unfortunately available only in some areas, presumably depending on local availability of charitable funding.[7] It offers counselling to children and young people experiencing difficulties as a result of parental separation, divorce or reconstituted families.

➤ *Bereavement services* specifically for children may be available in some areas through Winston's Wish,[8] or CRUSE.[9]

➤ *Local or national support groups* may be an invaluable source of support for carers of children with common conditions such as ADHD or rare conditions such as Duchenne muscular dystrophy.

Many of these agencies will take self-referrals from the young person or a carer; some prefer this.

SUMMARY
Referral to a specialist agency is more than just writing a quick note. The more preparation and care is taken in not only writing the referral, but also preparing the child and carers, the more likely it is to achieve something.

RESOURCES: WEBSITES PROVIDING A WEALTH OF INFORMATION
- www.youngminds.org.uk
- www.chimat.org.uk/camhs
- www.camh.org.uk

REFERENCES

1 Young Minds. *What are Child and Adolescent Mental Health Services?* London: Young Minds; 2006. Free to download from: www.dawsonmarketing.co.uk/youngminds/shop (accessed 6 April 2011).

2 Thorpe H, Dugmore O, Elliott HM. *CAMHS Inside Out: a young person's guide to child and adolescent mental health services.* London: Royal College of Psychiatrists (QINMAC: Quality Improvement Network for Multi-Agency CAMHS); 2009.

3 CAMHS Evidence-Based Practice Unit. *Choosing What's Best For You.* London: University College, London; 2007. Available at: www.ucl.ac.uk/clinical-psychology/EBPU/publications/children.php (accessed 6 April 2011).

4 www.education.gov.uk/childrenandyoungpeople/strategy/integratedworking/caf/a0068957/the-caf-process

5 www.nspcc.org.uk

6 www.direct.gov.uk/en/YoungPeople/index.htm

7 www.relate.org.uk

8 www.winstonswish.org.uk

9 www.crusebereavementcare.org.uk

Index